"This book expertly combines the authors' solution-focused perspectives and academic working in the fresh air, add solution-focused your adventures with clients, it's a must read and a book to go back to again and again."

Mark McKergow, PhD, author of *The Next Generation of Solution-Focused Practice*

"An eminently practical book of strategies for creating better lives outside of the consulting room."

Scott D. Miller, PhD, founder of the International Center for Clinical Excellence and coauthor of *Better Results: Using Deliberate Practice to Improve Your Therapeutic Effectiveness*

"The field needs the voices of Will and Stephan, who pull together the past and present uses of solution-focused therapy to engage the current and future generations of practitioners. This book can help practitioners resist the pull of 'curing the disease' and embrace an understanding of how clients possess solutions they have yet to discover."

From the foreword by H. Lee Gillis, APA's 2020 Arthur Teicher Group Psychologist of the Year

"In this pioneering book, Will Dobud and Stephan Natynczuk invite us into their adventure of taking solution-focused practice outdoors and show convincingly that it belongs there. If you ever work in an outdoor setting, or are contemplating doing so, I recommend putting this in your backpack and joining them."

Guy Shennan, therapist, consultant, trainer, and author of *Solution-Focused Practice: Effective Communication to Facilitate Change*

"Looking for a textbook that will enhance your therapeutic work outdoors? Here it is! The authors' skillful provision of a solution-focused and hands-on model for outdoor and adventure therapy is not only written in an accessible and down-to-earth manner, it is also conveyed in a heartfelt and inspirational way. I am deeply moved by their beautiful references to clients throughout the book as everything from superheroes to sunsets, whilst reiterating their rightful position as co-adventurers for change."

Carina Ribe Fernee, PhD, co-chair of the Adventure Therapy International Committee and clinician and researcher in the Department of Child and Adolescent Mental Health at Sørlandet Hospital in Norway

"Science has proved that a patient can heal faster and require fewer pain killers if they are able to see a tree outside their window. How much more can the mind and body heal, destress, and strengthen in close connection with the natural world? Will Dobud and Stephan Natynczuk have given us the gift of a road map, a work of research destined to become the bible of and a practical guide to effecting outdoor therapy of all kinds."

Les Stroud, creator of the survival TV genre (with *Survivorman*) and author of *Survive: Essential Skills and Tactics to Get You Out of Anywhere Alive*

Solution-Focused Practice in Outdoor Therapy

Solution-Focused Practice in Outdoor Therapy presents a comprehensive model for working therapeutically with clients outdoors, with adventure, and in any outdoor setting – from a typical one-hour session to multi-day expeditions.

Chapters lay out a robust and pragmatic model for opening the counseling room door using solution-focused methods. Dobud and Natynczuk bring together research on best practice in psychotherapy, monitoring therapeutic outcomes, safe and inclusive leadership, supervision, and self-care to present a robust framework for working therapeutically outdoors. Case vignettes are presented throughout the book, and a field manual is available for free download with purchase of the book.

Will W. Dobud, PhD, MSW, is a social work lecturer with Charles Sturt University and has been involved in outdoor therapy in the United States, Australia, and Norway. His internationally recognized research focuses on participant experiences in care and improving outcomes in the outdoor therapies.

Stephan Natynczuk, DPhil, MBA, LPIOL, FRSA, MNCS(accred), has been professionally involved in experiential education since 1988. Stephan enjoys training aspirant outdoor practitioners internationally and runs a private outdoor therapy practice. His research focuses on effective practice and professionalism in outdoor therapy.

Solution-Focused Practice in Outdoor Therapy

Co-Adventuring for Change

Will W. Dobud
and Stephan Natynczuk

Routledge
Taylor & Francis Group

NEW YORK AND LONDON

Cover image: © Getty Images

First published 2023
by Routledge
605 Third Avenue, New York, NY 10158

and by Routledge
4 Park Square, Milton Park, Abingdon, Oxon, OX14 4RN

Routledge is an imprint of the Taylor & Francis Group, an informa business

© 2023 Will W. Dobud and Stephan Natynczuk

Library of Congress Cataloging-in-Publication Data
Names: Dobud, Will W., author. | Natynczuk, Stephan, author.
Title: Solution-focused practice in outdoor therapy : co-adventuring for change / Will W. Dobud, Stephan Natynczuk.
Description: New York, NY : Routledge, 2023. | Includes bibliographical references and index. |
Identifiers: LCCN 2022007513 (print) | LCCN 2022007514 (ebook) | ISBN 9781032108803 (hardback) | ISBN 9781032108810 (paperback) | ISBN 9781003217558 (ebook)
Subjects: LCSH: Adventure therapy. | Nature--Therapeutic use. |
Solution-focused therapy. | Brief psychotherapy. | Evidence-based psychotherapy.
Classification: LCC RC489.A38 D63 2023 (print) | LCC RC489.A38 (ebook) | DDC 616.89/147--dc23/eng/20220622
LC record available at https://lccn.loc.gov/2022007513
LC ebook record available at https://lccn.loc.gov/2022007514

ISBN: 978-1-032-10880-3 (hbk)
ISBN: 978-1-032-10881-0 (pbk)
ISBN: 978-1-003-21755-8 (ebk)

DOI: 10.4324/9781003217558

Typeset in Goudy
by SPi Technologies India Pvt Ltd (Straive)

Access the Support Material: www.routledge.com/9781032108810

Contents

To Our Dearest Adventurous Reader

We wrote this book with you in mind. We hope you are a curious person exploring how to be at your best in your work, which is, we guess, being helpful to others who are looking for change in their lives. Perhaps they, and maybe you, are stuck in how to resolve a certain challenge. Of course, that is not inevitable. While you are looking for a way to be helpful, they cannot see a way out of their situation. The approach we talk about here takes your co-adventurers to a future time when whatever brought them to consult you, whatever their "problem" was, no longer exists. Our practice is about co-adventuring. While we do engage in useful conversations – co-facilitated conversations – this work is nothing more than a shared experience with future-focused questions to help co-adventurers bring about change for themselves

We hope you enjoy our offering: we have tried to be at our best as writers. We kept writing until the nice person at Routledge said our time was up and we should put down our pens. There is more we could have added, though we had to stop. We hope that there is enough here to be getting on with for now. We have tried to navigate between helpful, accurate anecdotes, and academic writing to make this an enjoyable and thoughtful read in every way. You, of course, will decide that and we appreciate all feedback. Our hope is that we can tell you of our work, which is both fun and helpful for our co-adventurers, who some might refer to as clients, patients, participants, or service users. They are, of course, the most important people in this work and so we dedicate our work and this book to all of them.

With the warmest of regards,

Will & Stephan, two very good friends,
very similar yet geographically oceans apart.

Foreword

H. Lee Gillis

I have worked in, written about, and taught adventure therapy since the 1970s. In the mid-1980s, a student in my doctoral program told me of a psychotherapy workshop he recently attended that focused on solutions more than problems. The student shared an example he heard of working with someone who wanted to stop smoking cigarettes. Instead of coming up with strategies to target reducing his smoking behavior, the workshop focused on exploring all the times he did not smoke during the day. How could these moments be increased? Instead of a problem-focus (time spent smoking), could there be a solution-focus (time spent not smoking)? Instead of finding problems, could the mindset become finding solutions amongst what the client was already doing? I was intrigued.

I attempted to incorporate a solution-focused mindset and fought the urge to identify and treat the problem/disease. Together with my friend and colleague Dr. Michael Gass, I wrote articles in the mid-1990s and presented on a solution-focus at regional and national conferences to practitioners engaged primarily in adventure activities with a therapeutic message. I always like the image of the glass with water up to the midpoint. Water is a solution. The challenge of the half-full or half-empty glass was what comes next? Do you help the client discover how to fill their glass full by adding new techniques or practices, or do you focus on the solution in the glass and inquire what the client did to fill the glass to where it was? Could the knowledge, skills, and abilities within the client be engaged? Could therapy in the outdoors be the catalyst?

This book goes well beyond what Dr. Gass and I were doing at the time. The field needs the voices of Will and Stephan, who pull together the past and present uses of solution-focused therapy to engage the current and future generations of practitioners. This book can help practitioners resist the pull of "curing the disease" and embrace an understanding of how clients possess solutions they have yet to discover.

Drink up!

H. L. (Lee) Gillis, PhD, ABPP

www.researchgate.net/profile/H-L-lee-Gillis

Professor of Psychology

Chair: Department of Psychological Science

Licensed Psychologist #1335(GA)

Board Certified in Group Psychology

Certified Clinical Adventure Therapist

Georgia College Milledgeville, GA 31061

The Great Horse Manure Crisis of 1894: A Shitty Preface

"In 50 years, every street in London will be buried under nine feet of manure," *The Times* predicted in 1894. This was a problem not unique to London. New York, Paris, and other major cities were also "drowning in horse manure." New York, for example, had a population of at least 150,000 horses, each of which produced between 15 and 35 pounds (roughly 7 to 16 kilograms) of manure per day. An uncomfortable buzz of flies came as horse manure piled up in the streets and when the manure dried, it was blown everywhere in the wind.

In 1898, the crisis led to the first international urban-planning conference in the Big Apple. City planners from all over the world attended the New York conference as horse manure was burying all major nineteenth century cities alive. With no exaggeration, the future of urban civilization hung in the balance. The conference, scheduled for ten days, was abandoned after three. According to Davies (2004), "None of the delegates could see any solution to the growing crisis posed by urban horses and their output" (para. 7).

During this time, Henry Ford was perfecting his Model T and designing an assembly line to accelerate the production of motor vehicles. Trains made for faster travel than horses since Stevenson's Rocket won the Rainhill Trials in 1829. Horse drawn cabs were quickly replaced with electric trams and auto-buses. By 1912, the problem no city planner could solve in 1898 was no longer such a problem. The solution held little relation to the problem everyone faced.

This solution, though life-saving at the time, came with its clear side effects. The current climate crisis is obviously now of great concern and has yet to become manageable. It is something we have witnessed firsthand in our experience adventuring in the outdoors as the environments and habitats we frequent become noticeably different. Seasons are not quite so regular, and the extremes of weather are much harsher.

The great horse manure crisis of 1894 (Davies, 2004) is used in economics, history, and business studies as a metaphor for problem solving, so we, of course, found it a useful preamble to this book and metaphor for co-constructing solutions with clients. After all, any metaphor about "horse shit" is a good one for us as we search for an efficient, effective, and robust model for encouraging the helping professions to open their doors and embrace the great outdoors. The solutions people use to tackle life's obstacles do not need to be related to the problem. Focusing on the problem is likely to lead to more problem talk, and mostly keeps the problem alive.

This text is about adopting solution-focused brief therapy in the outdoors; an approach with proven robustness in its simplicity and efficiency in terms of bringing about significant change in minimum time. This is an adaptable practice blending talking therapy, coaching, mentoring, and leadership with the intrinsic therapeutic qualities on offer in the outdoors. We also give much attention to how practitioners can strive to be their best.

About the Authors

Will W. Dobud In 2008, or 09, not too sure, I sat through a full day's work-shop presented by Matthew Selekman at a National Association of Social Workers' conference in Baltimore, Maryland. I was urged to attend by my then boss and supervisor and most inspirational mentor, Brooke Brody. Just after our lunch break, I shot back to the University of Maryland–Baltimore County for an exam required as part of my Bachelor of Social Work degree. I rushed so as to catch the conclusion of Matthew Selekman's training and was left in awe. The focus on solutions and creativity, at least to me, ap-peared to work seamlessly in my outdoor therapy practice. The workshop concluded and while preparing for the dreaded drive down I-95 in peak traf-fic, I saw Matthew Selekman sitting at the bus stop. I drove up, lowered the window, and asked if he would like a lift to Baltimore–Washington Interna-tional Airport. He hopped in my car, a small four-wheel drive with a cracked windscreen full of caving equipment and a grab bag of outdoor gear. It was this day that I was forever entrenched in adapting solution-focused practice to the outdoors.

Since then, I moved to Australia, continued my social work studies, and completed a PhD focused on people's experiences in outdoor therapy. This book has been a dream of mine and meeting Dr. Stephan Natynczuk and slowly imprinting our thoughts on paper has been nothing but rewarding.

Stephan Natynczuk Apparently I was a solution-focused practitioner before I knew solution-focused practice even existed. This was pointed out to me by a friend and colleague, Jeff Matthews, who was studying for a Masters in Solution-Focused Practice. When we met up after a few years, we were talk-ing about our work and what informed our practice. Mine was very eclectic, drawing on my scientific research in behavioral ecology especially around signals and choices, Rogerian humanism, some existential philosophy, some pedagogy with respect to adventure and experiential learning outdoors, some Zen, assorted philosophies, and lots more. "You know what you're doing don't you?" said Jeff. "It's solution-focused." I had more to learn and I enrolled in a series of courses and training with some of the most prominent solution-focused thinkers and practitioners through BRIEF in London, UK. In turn, I too became a trainer in solution-focused practice, specializing in working outdoors with youth in crisis through adventure.

For most of my 30 plus years of professional practice, I have mostly worked with young people, co-adventuring underground, on mountains, rivers, and lakes, in forests, and all with solution-focused conversations. Usually working one to one with an assistant as safety back up, I have worked with more than a thousand co-adventurers in a solution-focused way. Recently, I have branched out into training and supervising practitioners. I thoroughly enjoy that work, too. Much of my experience and learning is presented in this book, which has been an absolute pleasure to write with Will.

Part I
Co-Adventuring for Change

1
Co-Adventuring for Change

"The therapist is a co-adventurer, exploring the landscape and encountering multiple vantage points while crossing the terrain of the client's theory of change. When stuck along the way, we join clients in looking for and exploring alternate routes on their own maps. In the process clients uncover trails we never dreamed existed."

Duncan et al. (2011, p. 136)

I (Will) had a client, Oscar, who once said to me, "I should present at an adventure therapy conference." We were hiking during a session, and he knew I was traveling to a conference the following week. Those events were something I enjoyed, and he knew it. After all, if you have any chance in your lifetime to attend an adventure, wilderness, bush, or outdoor therapy conference, you will be hard pressed to find such a fun, engaging group of individuals to play with. That said, I asked what he would present. He told me, "You adventure therapists just place the word 'therapy' after 'adventure' to have fun while calling it work." He stressed that hanging out with "cool" people made the therapy more enjoyable. He was not wrong. Throughout our work together, we had done just about every adventurous activity under the sun: canoeing, hiking, fishing, climbing, snorkeling, caving, mountain biking; he even attended a few of my 14-day expeditions.

Though I certainly enjoyed our time together, important things happened. Diagnosed with autism spectrum disorder in primary school, Oscar struggled early in his education. Thus, his parents elected to home school. Oscar was particularly sensitive to fluorescent lighting and every therapist's office and school setting left him in a state of sensory overload. Raised in a rural environment, he spent the majority of his time outdoors. Catching reptiles, fishing, and foraging for wild mushrooms were some of his many hobbies. He repeatedly wanted to join the local scouts group, but left each attempt demoralized from the bullying.

DOI: 10.4324/9781003217558-2

One year, bush fires forced his family to take refuge in a relative's home, their rural property reduced to ash. This time of change hit Oscar particularly hard. His mother called my office saying she had a son struggling to adapt with the recent changes and family stress. What stood out was that Oscar wanted a therapist to work with him outdoors. "He actually wants an outdoor therapist?" I asked. I did not see many young people eager to see any type of therapist, let alone one willing to take their work outside!

Funded by Australia's National Disability Insurance Scheme, Oscar's family were fortunate to have adequate third party reimbursement to cover many of our adventures. Of course, case managers wanted goals and measurable outcomes; as most funders do. I checked some of his case notes and found the usual clichéd goals. Regulate anxiety. We can work on that. Create an education plan. We can do that too. Still, I asked Oscar and his family about their best hopes for our work together.

Fast forward a few weeks, Oscar's mother called to say how much her son loved our adventures. Things were progressing smoothly. Everyone was happy with the service provided. Oscar was handling anxious experiences better, such as living with his extended family while the bushfires were extinguished, and he felt welcomed to a new scout group. We began adding more time between our sessions. Oscar would email me every five or six weeks. The emails were blunt and straight to the point. "Fishing. Thursday? Want to talk."

"Sure," I would reply. "What time?"

As each session came to an end, I asked something along the lines of, "What can you take away from this session that can help you through the week?"

"This," he responded. He described how he feels relaxed when doing things outdoors and found our conversations useful. There was something different happening in the moment to contrast the stresses at home.

Before what would be his 11th grade, Oscar expressed the desire to return to mainstream public school. While I still saw Oscar every few months, which was part of his government funded treatment plan, I did not expect to hear this. His family voiced apprehension. How was he going to handle the social setting, let alone the workload? What about the lighting? Still, Oscar's parents listened, enrolled him in the local public school, and he started attending. Before the second term, Oscar was nominated to become a prefect, a senior role in the school community, typically elected by his peers and teachers. Oscar's parents and I could not help but shrug our shoulders and laugh with joy at the appointment.

Before the senior students were entering their mid-year exams, Oscar was seen by a school counselor telling the students to spend time outside before the exams. He told them it helps with restoration and stress reduction. "Maybe he *should* present at the conference," I thought. He eventually became the school's *Prefect of Wellbeing* – a fitting title that would certainly give him some credibility to present at an adventure therapy conference.

Now in his 20s, Oscar eventually graduated from high school and is no longer a therapy client. After all, this is a "brief" therapy technique we are talking about, and he was an exception given the amount of adventures we enjoyed together, which he always scheduled himself. Oscar typically attends my 14-day expeditions as a mentor. This experience helps him complete outdoor recreation certificates, which aids in his employability through vocational training areas such as workplace safety and safe food handling. He wants to be a guide and do similar outdoor work. He is good at it.

Oscar catches up with me every now and then when he is back visiting his family. On a recent canoe trip, I asked him what made our work together meaningful. He talked about how when we were mountain biking or fishing, both undertakings at which he is naturally skilled, I never took the role of expert. He told me he preferred to just do things together as equals. Of course, there is no equal therapeutic relationship, but he was tired of people telling him which meditation app to download and the overkill teaching of social skills, like maintaining eye contact. He was already doing these things well enough and did not find those interventions useful. While honored by the praise, I spent just six to seven hours a year with Oscar, including times on expedition. It is hard to take credit for his progress.

Oscar's mother was an incredible stakeholder; one so many clinicians and teachers neglected. She helped Oscar with so many social skills throughout his childhood that I knew those areas did not require my attention. No previous therapist had recognized the valued resource she was. In fact, she is returning to university where she will study teaching. Her hope is to work with young people with learning disabilities – a role she is already skilled at and sees her at her best.

Of course, this was an "easy" case. The young person showed up wanting something in particular: outdoor therapy. I listened, and we did what he hoped we would. I listened to his parents and funders with what they wanted as well. His case managers took note and referred more of their youngsters. Like all therapeutic endeavors, some cases went seamlessly like this one. Others had their ups and downs.

After presenting such a narrative, full of ripe therapeutic context and wonderful descriptions of change, we find it important to make explicitly clear that we are not interested in presenting "solution-focused therapy in the outdoors" as some new approach. We are not here to claim this approach is any better than the next. There are over 600 brands of psychotherapy, probably 1,000 (Meichenbaum & Lilienfeld, 2018), and all tend to work equally well (Miller et al., 2013; Wampold & Imel, 2015). We hope readers will realize throughout this book, and particularly our discussion in Part III, that simply flipping through these pages or grasping the context is, unfortunately, not likely to impact your outcomes. We need to work hard on our practice, to increase our attention to the fine details of what we can improve, and practice these areas deliberately. With that said, a clear mission statement is presented in the following section, which encompasses a clear, effective, robust, evidenced model for taking therapy to the outdoors. We provide a specific and concrete model to counter the messy and, at times, disorganized world of outdoor therapies (Dobud & Cavanaugh, 2020). This is a necessary step in the right direction for the outdoor therapies, and hopefully others follow with presenting their own evidence-informed approaches.

Mission Statement: Making the Outdoors Count

There are numerous models of outdoor therapies and even more names for this type of therapy. In a recent edited collection, outdoor therapy approaches included *wilderness therapy*, *adventure therapy*, *bush adventure therapy*, *nature-based therapy*, *forest therapy*, *surf therapy*, and *horticulture therapy*, among others (Harper & Dobud, 2020). Within these approaches were references to cognitive-behavioral, narrative, psychodynamic, solution-focused, trauma-informed, acceptance and commitment, and gestalt therapies; just to name a few of the many theoretical orientations informing this wonderfully diverse field. While varying in names and perspectives, the structures of these models are entirely different within themselves.

Some outdoor practitioners, for example, provide the typical one-hour psychotherapy session around an exercise outdoors, others real open-ended adventure-based explorations, while others deliver a series of day-long endeavors. Those working in expedition or residential settings could run multi-day or even multi-month programs. When it comes to defining what we do, it is too easy to stick with generic descriptions of our work. We have published using terms like adventure or wilderness therapy, and this, we argue, is often due to simplicity (Harper et al., 2019).

For example, it would be a mouthful to refer to our work as *Feedback-Informed Solution-Focused Brief Adventure Therapy*. Add to this the range of outdoor settings used in practices. Many outdoor practitioners will resonate with operating in near-by nature, or remote wilderness settings, or even a local garden or parkland (Harper et al., 2019). Our mission with this book is to present just one bona-fide, evidence-informed model for taking our therapeutic practices into these wonderful environments, no matter how they appear or how far they exist from urban settings. If you are already working intentionally outside, this book will provide, foremost, evidence-based strategies for not only guiding your approach, but embracing the available empirical research to improve your clients' experiences and outcomes in outdoor therapy.

We stand on the shoulders of our colleagues, many of them friends, and do not intend to discredit the work cited or communicate previous work as inadequate. While we agree with most, we struggle with the ethics of some. This book was not written to cut the heels of those aiming to push our field forward. Books, such as Gass et al. (2012, 2020), Harper et al. (2019) and Harper and Dobud (2020), are emerging with increasing frequency, and all add to the wider understanding of the amazing opportunities our field offers for meaningful and useful change.

Our book presents a very specific, pragmatic, and intentional model of therapy and examines its use in the outdoors. The differences between the outdoor therapies are razor thin. Taking therapy outside works and works well (Bowen & Neill, 2013). Our text examines a robust and labeled framework for facilitating useful therapeutic conversations in outdoor settings which efficiently and effectively co-constructs helpful change as we host and co-adventure in nature.

This introductory chapter will provide some background and context to solution-focused brief therapy and clinical practice in the outdoors. We present some of the history of solution-focused approaches and its evolution. We argue that a solution focused framework was influential for early approaches to the adventure-based therapies. However, these ideas were eclipsed by more problem-focused ideas that were influenced by a medical model (diagnosis requirement, focus on treatment and cure, etc.) and the economic and political forces of the evidence-based practice paradigm. Each following section introduces, defines, and presents some of the key evolutions of solution-focused brief therapy and the theoretical underpinnings informing this work. Those chapters following examine how we position outdoor therapies among the many different available models for helping and how we refer to those we work with.

Thinking Outside the ~~Box~~ Counseling Room

Outdoor therapies are often considered the *alternative* to the much more normal and popular talking therapies. For the past decade, researchers, practitioners, and advocates have fought tirelessly to show policymakers, insurance companies, and funders the promise of therapy outdoors (e.g. Norton et al., 2014). What has come of this, in our opinion, is an unjustified attempt to achieve superiority over therapy indoors. As described in Chapter 2, the goal of supremacy as a model for psychotherapy, while ambitious, has led to many new treatments, yet no improvements in psychotherapy outcomes (Harper, 2009). However, before unpacking this, we must consider how those regulating and gatekeeping therapy think.

Despite all the misfortune, loss, and economic hardship caused by the COVID-19 pandemic, therapists were taught a valuable lesson. During the many international lockdowns, therapists had two options: 1) adapt their work to online or telehealth modalities; or 2) go outside. Many quit their jobs as well. Third party payers did not care. In fact, virtual therapy or outdoor therapy became *safer* than sitting on the clinician's couch. What we learned was that where therapy occurs had almost zero impact on outcomes. For example, a recent meta-analysis by Fernandez et al. (2021) found:

> therapy is no less efficacious when delivered via videoconferencing than in-person… Live psychotherapy by video emerges not only as a popular and convenient choice but also one that is now upheld by meta-analytic evidence.
>
> (n.p.)

Dobud and Harper (2018) landed on the same finding, except with therapy conducted indoors or out. The concept of privileging one therapy setting over the next is certainly not an evidence-based one. Neither is the decision not to position online or outdoor therapy as equally accessible to the office or couch. Ample evidence has demonstrated this privilege does not exist. As we have learned to adapt our lives to new normals and renegotiated our relationship to work and life, we hope that the idea of what a counseling room looks like can be within that new normal. We hope that return does not involve regulated and necessitated indoor therapy. We prefer to have options on the table for people to consider when seeking therapeutic support. Whether it is online, the couch, or the great outdoors is no matter to us. We are simply among the many doing this work outside.

Who We Work With

Language and terminology are important, and we are frequently asked how we should label those we work with. Are they clients, patients, participants, service-users, consumers, customers, co-adventurers, or simply just people? If this topic is one of your passions, reflect on what feels right for you and consider how your decision is likely to impact your work. That said, this is a therapy book, and we had to settle for something to help differentiate our co-workers from those receiving the outdoor therapy service. For the purposes of our book, there are some important philosophical assumptions informing our decision.

Our first preference is co-adventurers, as Duncan et al. (2011) referred to in the quote we used to begin this chapter. Not only does it link with the co-construction philosophical underpinnings of solution-focused practice (discussed further in Chapters 3 and 4), it emphasizes people's *active participation*. Thus, "participant" works too. After all, they are *participating* in the outdoor therapy experience. "Consumers" could work as we do consider our work consumer-oriented. We also have no problem with the word client, but focus on their personhood first. The word patient seems too passive, and customers too capitalistic and neo-liberal. "Service users" may sound like a service done *to* or *for* someone, passive rather than actively done together. We know countries with Latin roots may prefer to use patients. Cultural context matters. There is a lot to consider.

You will notice throughout this book that co-adventurer, participant, and client are used somewhat interchangeably. This is not meant to confuse the reader, and it is never this simple. The people who take on one of our many adventures have rich histories. When we talk about the assumptions, techniques, and questions used in our practice, we will use these terms. It is not our intention to position the people we work with as passive recipients of our clinical expertise, nor are they homogenous in culture, experience, gender, sexual identity, geographic origin, or any other classification. Quite the contrary. We do, however, require some distinction, and we feel ethically content with how we have honored the richness and participation of the incredible co-adventurers, participants, and clients we have experienced this work with. Of course, pseudonyms are provided and care is taken to maintain the confidentiality and privacy of the co-adventurers. Many of the case vignettes contained within this book come from years of outdoor therapy practice and consultancy work with various organizations.

One final consideration before moving on, and we are probably nit picking here – the people we work with are never *our* clients in the sense that they belong to us, that we know best what they need. Practitioners strive to reduce the inherent power differential that naturally occurs between the helper and the helped. It feels odd to appropriate ownership over another person, especially one experiencing disadvantage and vulnerability, and not right to claim their successes as our own. Our focus is on what we can do together and the meaning our co-adventurers construct from the experience.

Our Field Manual

In the back of this book you will notice a series of appendices we refer to as our *Field Manual for Solution-Focused Practice Outdoors* (see Appendix A). This is a series of worksheets, solution-focused questions, useful tools for soliciting client feedback, and considerations for supervision. At first, we aimed to produce the manual as a separate text; something spiral bound and printed on waterproof paper you could take with you on your next outdoor therapy session. But we did not want you to have to break your wallet. Instead, it is printed in the back of this text and available online as a PDF.

We will reference specific areas of the field manual throughout. For best use, we recommend printing the PDF from our book's site and laminating the pages. For example, when conducting program evaluations outdoors, we have printed a copy of our outcome measures, laminated them, and let our co-adventurers use dry erase markers to complete them. This way we can collect the data, record them in our notes, and wipe clean the measures for the next person to use. Not only does this reduce waste, it is less weight to carry.

When participants have drifted off to sleep during an expedition, our group of practitioners might join around a fire for a processing of the day. To remain solution-focused, we use the guide available in the field manual. We hope you find this brief resource useful in adopting this evidence-informed approach to outdoor therapy.

The remainder of this chapter introduces solution-focused practice, its intersection with therapy outdoors, and provides our initial assumptions for approaching this work. We touch on our concerns with the medical model and its influence in how we conceptualize and fund various therapy services.

Introducing Solution-Focused Brief Therapy

Solution-focused brief therapy was "born" in the late 1970s at the Brief Family Therapy Center (BFTC), an inner-city outpatient mental health service in Milwaukee, Wisconsin, by Steve de Shazer and Insoo Kim Berg (1997). Developing the earlier work from the Mental Research Institute, Palo Alto (Weakland et al., 1974), de Shazor and Berg spent a good deal of their time watching thousands of hours of therapy sessions, the work focused on simply answering one question: *What works, and how can practitioners get better at doing it?* While observing therapy sessions, observers were "Carefully noting the questions, behaviors, and emotions that led to clients conceptualizing and achieving viable, real-life solutions" (de Shazer et al., 2012, p. 1). As solution-focused work developed, its recognition surrounded a series of techniques, like the popular miracle and scaling questions (Berg & Dolan, 2001). For us, common practice includes the use of "simple-to-ask future-focused questions" (Natynczuk, 2014, p. 26) with further detail evoked by asking clients what difference aspects of that preferred future will make. We work with the client to find examples of moments where they have enacted aspects of their preferred future previously.

McKergow (2016) argued that much of solution-focused practice and literature has grown since the original conceptions of Steve de Shazer, Insoo Kim Berg, and colleagues. Practice has evolved and simplified. Quite an achievement given de Shazer's insistence that "there is no orthodoxy" in solution-focused approaches. Still, McKergow (2016) argued that distinctions are still necessary in order to keep practice from becoming muddled, which we agree is one of our motivations for writing this book with outdoor practice firmly in mind.

Since the days of Berg and de Shazer (de Shazer, 1984; de Shazer & Berg, 1997), the evolution of solution-focused brief therapy continued and empirical support developed further. In a review of the effectiveness of solution-focused approaches, Bond et al. (2013) found that although the available research is limited by few high-quality studies, as rated for methodological appropriateness, the evidence from these studies supported the efficacy of solution-focused approaches for "moderate levels of internalizing and externalizing behavior difficulties" (p. 721). Of the 38 studies included in their synthesis, a solution-focus was effective for *increasing* hope, self-efficacy, coping skills, family relationships, confidence, goal attainment, self-esteem, self-image, social adjustment, and social competence, and *decreasing* depressive symptoms, school dropout rates, post-traumatic symptoms, complaints, cognitive difficulties, anti-social attitudes, aggression, truancy rates, and behavior difficulties. Though positive, the authors warned readers to be cautious with their findings.

Many of the studies included in Bond et al.'s (2013) review compared solution-focused interventions to no-treatment or placebo control groups. In a nutshell, this means that half the research participants received an effective helping modality while the other half received nothing or treatments designed to be inherently ineffective (Frank & Frank, 1991). When solution-focused approaches were compared to conditions where therapists provided a therapy designed to be equally helpful, there was little to no difference in outcomes (Adams et al., 1991; Yarbrough & Thompson, 2002). This finding is not unique to solution-focused or any other therapy. Miller et al. (2008) found the equivalency in specific treatments for youth mental disorders. In meta-analyzing the direct comparison trials for the treatment of post-traumatic stress disorder, Wampold et al. (2010) also found all therapies to be equally efficacious. As mentioned above, Dobud and Harper (2018) found no study to show outdoor or adventurous approaches to therapy more effective than its comparison groups that could not be confirmed by methodological issues, such as non-equivocal treatment groups. In the following chapter, we dive deeper into these issues and present some of the most replicated findings to help practitioners inform their helping approach based on the best available evidence we could find at the time of writing.

Solution-focused brief therapy has a rich history drawing on an adamant stance centered on a clients' best hopes and preferred future. Much of the focus was on how to be as efficient as possible when working therapeutically with people in distress. Doing anything unlikely to contribute to outcome or client progress is inconsequential. We are reminded of William of Ockham's postulation in 1344 that "What can be done with fewer means is done in vain with many" (Shennan, 2019). Famously becoming known as *Ockham's Razor*, this call to simplify practice shaped the solution-focused therapy taught to me (Stephan) and others at BRIEF (Ratner et al., 2012). It is a useful guiding principle for many things in life. Keep it simple. Do more of what is working, and throw away what is not. Nothing more, nothing less. Not one session, hour, or day too many. Colloquially, people could have better things to do.

We were interested to see that solution-focused assumptions are nothing new to outdoor and adventure-based therapies. We do, however, question where they move in favor of more complex, diagnostic adaptations. In the following section, we present some of the historical context, mostly informed by the works of Michael Gass and Lee Gillis in the early to mid-1990s. Additionally,

Walsh and Golins' (1976) exploration of the Outward Bound process contains many associations to solution-focused practice, such as privileging a person's self-determination, experiential processing, and embracing the core Rogerian conditions of change, though we are hard pressed to find any modality ignoring Roger's contribution.

Solution-Focus in Outdoor Therapies

As the popularity and research evidence for Outward Bound grew in the United States, Walsh and Golins (1976) conceptualized how this specific process led to change. Originally, the authors described a *motivated learner* engaging with a *unique physical* and *social environment*. That motivated learner then engages with a *characteristic set of problem-solving tasks* and experiences a *state of adapted dissonance*. As the learners adapt, they experience a sense of *mastery*, which *reorganizes the meaning and direction of the learner's experience*.

There are a few ways we use this description to inform our view of taking a solution-focus to outdoor settings, and these major assumptions will be examined further in Chapter 3. First, we view all our co-adventurers as motivated by something; curiosity is a basic mammalian behavior. Additionally, any therapy or counseling setting, indoors or out, *is* a unique physical and social environment. Walking into a stranger's office with diplomas nailed to the wall and an expansive bookshelf is certainly a novel setting. We venture away from Walsh and Golins (1976) in the prescribed problem-solving tasks and state of dissonance. Problem-solving tasks, like learning to make a fire by friction, may lead to a contraction of meaning: though it is the solution-focused conversation that is the intervention. This is when the participant, the co-adventurer, starts becoming cognitively active in their own change process. In this case, we argue practitioners should avoid focusing on simply learning a plethora of activities or games to prescribe to their clients, and instead develop their interpersonal, observational, and listening skills, and relentlessly kind curiosity.

For example, expedition-based outdoor therapy, such as residential wilderness therapy expeditions, may prescribe a series of tasks for an adolescent participant to complete in order to progress in the program (Dobud, 2020). While we have certainly witnessed our fair share of young people who find this approach useful, the rigid nature of such programming leads some youth to focus more on crossing items off their "therapy checklist." The danger is that this leads to *compliance*. Your client's focus is achieving what you set out for them in order to reach the next phase of their treatment. Behind the veil of achievement is a client focused on compliance. Compliance is not a therapeutic outcome.

What is essential to our work, and where we find Walsh and Golins' (1976) original conceptualization so useful, is the stressing of mastery. We have built on this notion to call our therapeutic setting a *Climate of Competence*. For our work to be effective, clients must feel they are at their best and have agency for the changes they need. We are not interested in defining what competence/mastery is for another person. For example, a couple on a marriage therapy retreat could fall gently backwards into a snowbank while gazing towards the stars. This could provide a sense of awe, togetherness, and understanding of each other, something their relationship lacked prior to the outdoor therapy. A young adolescent may benefit more from successfully scaling a rock wall or simply engaging appropriately with her schoolmates. We do not define mastery. It is experienced and constructed based on a person's interaction with the practitioner, the environment, and the social network involved. Change is solely owned by the client.

Nearly 20 years after Walsh and Golins' (1976) conceptualization, Gass and Gillis (1995) recognized solution-focused thinking as key to the change process within adventure therapy. They argued for practitioners to adopt a "philosophical shift in approaching client issues" (p. 63). Rather than focusing on specific therapeutic methods or the intentional choosing of outdoor activities, they presented groups of assumptions. If anything, this book is simply the ongoing development of their original approach to client change. Their discussion, in line with solution-focused practice at that time, involved seeking exceptions to a person's problem narrative to explore what the client was doing during times when the presenting problem did not exist, or at least was not present. With information about these exceptions, the practitioner encourages the client to notice times when they had either solved this problem successfully in the past, or had sufficiently coped.

Three decades have passed since Gass and Gillis (1995) discussed these concepts and theoretical assumptions about how we view those we work with seem all but gone with the wind. In the same time, solution-focused practice has evolved significantly, especially through the work of Ratner et al. (2012) at BRIEF in London. A number of models have emerged that emphasize a range of solution-focused tools, though with practitioners acutely focusing on clients' best interests and preferred future.

In our field, most outdoor therapy research has taken a drastic turn towards a problem-focused deficit model, exploring how outcomes correlate with specific moderators, such as diagnostic criteria, presenting problems, and readiness for change (Clark et al., 2004; Tucker et al., 2014). This deficit model evolution has continued despite diagnoses telling us little about how change occurs, providing no correlation to specific lengths of stay in residential treatment, or demonstrating any reliability that therapists will provide the best approach for resolving a client's concern (Brown et al., 1999; Wampold & Imel, 2015). Additionally, since their article (Gass & Gillis, 1995), tragic events and poorly defined practice has impacted the public image of therapy outdoors, especially in the context of US wilderness therapy (Anderson, 2014). Numerous cases of abuse, neglect, and client death while participating in residential and wilderness therapy programs in the United States have influenced this image (GAO, 2007). For these reasons, we must consider what we mean by "therapy" and how we can put the medical model to rest. At least for the time being.

The "Medical Model" and What We Mean When We Talk about Therapy

When we talk about therapy, we mean something that brings about a change that a person wants for themselves. This change occurs through careful conversations: it is a talking therapy. This can be controversial in outdoor and adventure therapies, especially those adopting an approach with active bodily engagement or one focused on the treatment of complex trauma (Harper & Doherty, 2020; Pringle et al., 2021). The reason we use the word *therapy* and *talking therapy* is an important one. For Wampold and Imel (2015), therapy is defined as:

> a primarily interpersonal treatment that is a) based on psychological principles; b) involves a trained therapist and a client who is seeking help for a mental disorder, problem, or complaint; c) is intended by the therapist to be remedial for the client disorder, problem, or complaint; and d) is adapted or individualized for the particular client and his or her disorder, problem, or complaint.
>
> (p. 37)

We just happen to do this outdoors where there are other rich factors, such as physical enjoyment of exercise, shared experiences of endeavor, joint enterprise, collective success, shared meals, being in nature, and personal time for reflection (Harper & Dobud, 2020). We can witness our co-adventurers at their best, explore the richness of metaphors outdoor experiences bring, utilize the many opportunities for reflection and natural mindfulness, and use skillful listening and questioning to focus participants' thinking on improving (Natynczuk, 2021).

The subsequent chapter examines how practitioners can inform their practice based on the best available evidence on how therapy works, no matter their profession, qualification, or years of experience. There is a fundamental position that we adopt in our practice, and we have included a few words about the medical model here to provide a stark contrast to the approach we describe in this book. The distinction could not be stronger.

Borrowed from the notion of evidence-based medicine (Wampold & Imel, 2015), proponents of the medical model believe that an appropriate diagnosis will help a practitioner choose the correct treatment from a range of options. The practitioner focuses first on what Duncan (2014) referred to as The Killer D's: Diagnoses, Deficits, Disorders, Dysfunctions, Disabilities, Deficiencies. It is about collecting signs and symptoms, matching them to a syndrome, and then treating the syndrome with an empirically supported treatment to make the patient well again. Obviously, this approach works well pharmacologically and physiologically, though therapeutically is often known as the deficit model (Sparks et al., 2007), as it concentrates on what is perhaps missing rather than what we could have more of to make things better. It is usual for a patient to sign a consent form for a procedure done to them for their benefit. Occasionally, the therapy is given without the patient's consent. As solution-focused practitioners, we might question whose interest is satisfied by the treatment and if it is in any way solution-*forced* (Thomas, 2007). This occurs when a practitioner "fails to acknowledge (1) the client's painful story, (2) the client's view of what he/she considers an exception that makes a difference to him/her, and (3) the client's self-defined reasons for seeking therapy" (Nylund & Corsiglia, 1994, p. 5).

In opposition to the medical model, the practice we describe here is interested in nothing other than people's best interests, as they describe them to us. In a broad sense, solution-focused practice is non-normalizing and intensely client-centered. We ask clients what they want and how they would know when they have got something good enough. This is not a treatment done *to* people: it is an experience and outcome our client "does" for themselves. In fact, we strictly follow the solution-focused anecdote that the best practitioners receive fewer thank you notes than the others. A client perceives that they did the work themselves, which is consistent with Leave No Trace ethics practiced in caring for natural settings (Natynczuk & Dobud, 2021). We develop our discussion about Leave No Trace in Chapter 4.

Our role as practitioners is to listen carefully and ask questions to support people in unpacking their own preferred future. This demands trust. We trust people know what they want and they are the experts in their own lives.

We do not assume any privileged knowledge relating to those dreadful Killer D's. How could we know what is best for our client unless we ask and explore with collaborative curiosity? It is not for us to give unsolicited advice, to diagnose, to guess what is best through the lens of our own experiences, or attempt to *fix* people as any third person might deem best for them. We remain curious about a client's narrative, to trust them with what they say about their lives, and what they tell us they want to be different.

Whether to give advice or not can be problematic. On the one hand, are we negligent if we refuse to share information that could be to the client's advantage? Many of our professional bodies and codes of ethics would say so (Caldwell, 2015). On the other hand, we may set ourselves up to fail the client if the advice proves useless, even harmful, and our client blames us for making things worse. Within solution-focused practice, we might ask our client "Let's suppose you get the advice you need, what difference would that make to you?" We may perhaps say, "Another person I know was in a similar situation to the one you describe and this is what they did... How would you know if that worked for you too?" In essence, we avoid being responsible for a client's choice and encourage them to think things through for themselves, to foster their agency to make change, and to take responsibility for the choices they make to improve their situation. In essence, the client is their own intervention.

Rock climbers inherently get this. If you are supporting a climber from the ground, as the belayer, you are watching the climber's every move. You feel through the rope and listen attentively for requests for more or less slack. You watch closely and observe body language. The climber may ask for advice. You provide some ideas. "There is a foothold near your left knee, if that helps." Otherwise, you can encourage or remain silent should they power through the climb. If stuck along the route, we do not climb up next to them to chip away the rock to construct a new hand hold. This not only damages the natural environment, it takes away from the climber's journey. When the climber is successful and descends to the ground, we do not appropriate their success to anything we did. Sure, we were there for safety and helped to consider various strategies for success and mastery, yet it is their climb and they put the effort in. To think otherwise is to overinflate the role of the belayer, or therapy practitioner.

Though we examine the major implications for becoming an evidence-informed practitioner and the major themes for taking solution-focused practice to the outdoors, we use the remainder of this chapter to present the common tenets of the solution-focused practitioner. You will see as our approach develops that these ideas are deceptively simple. The skill is with listening and using a tool that builds on the answer thereby moving the client closer to their destination for the therapy. We hope you pocket these ideas, as we will expand on them in the coming chapters.

Tenets of Solution-Focused Practice

When I (Stephan) first trained as a counselor, I was struck by a rule of thumb: to "assume" made an "ass" out of "u" and "me." Ever since, I have remained wary of guessing what a client means in therapeutic conversations. I instead seek confirmation of what I do and do not understand. There are, however, a number of *assumptions* or principles that seem to be true in solution-focused practice (Selekman, 2005). Presented below are some of the assumptions we make about those we work with. While some of these may seem too mundane to matter, it is the rigidity and grounding in this stance that makes practicing this way so tempting.

What We Think about Clients
- Every person is unique.
- People come to us with resources and strengths, both personal and in their social networks.
- All clients have the ability to find their own solutions to the difficulties they have.
- One cannot change clients; they can only change themselves.
- The therapy practitioner is not the expert on the client or their social network; the client is.
- A client's own solution that fits their own situation is more likely to be implemented and maintained than something suggested to them.

What We Think about Problems
- No problem happens all the time: there are always exceptions that can be found and built upon.
- A focus on the possible and changeable is more helpful than a focus on the overwhelming and intractable.
- The client is not the problem. The problem is the problem.
- The problem and the solution occur in the interaction between people rather than residing within people.
- Problems that appear complex might not require a complex solution.

What We Think about Change

- Change is constant.
- Small changes can make a big difference.
- Rapid change or resolution can happen when people hit on ideas that work.
- Change is likely to occur sooner rather than later.
- There may have been some pre-session change.

What We Think about Practice

- Lasting change is more likely to happen when you find out what is working and help people focus on what happens when they do more of it.
- Change is happening all the time. Our job is to identify and amplify useful change.
- People are more likely to behave and/or think differently when you work with their ideas of useful change.

More important than the techniques utilized throughout this book are these tenets. We recommend printing these from the field manual (see Appendix) and using them to inform your discussion during a future supervision session, or while sitting around a fire talking with your colleagues when your co-adventurers are resting in their tents. They inform how we view those we work with and conceptualize what happens during an outdoor therapy session. When stuck, practitioners can revisit these ideas to construct a more useful assessment of what is occurring in the interaction.

A Concluding Invitation

Solution-focused approaches have been criticized for a range of issues. Critics argue the modality remains too shallow and ignores the macro structures in place which oppress, or that the therapy moves too fast to build strong therapeutic alliances with its recipients. We have heard many times: "I can't see this modality working with [insert oppressed population of your choice]." We invite you throughout this book to consider outdoor therapies from a different perspective, one in which co-adventurers are the heroes at the center of their own journey.

To think otherwise is to inflate the practitioner's role and stereotype our clients based on our theories of pathology. For instance, we have heard, "I like the miracle question, but would never use it with asylum seekers." A quick Google Scholar search brings up some interesting research projects about effective solution-focused practice with similar populations. "Solution-focused approaches do not take into account trauma." Based on the available research, solution-focused approaches have led to large, statistically significant improvements in post-traumatic growth (Eads & Yee Lee, 2019). Each of these statements includes an assumption about the person(s) seated across from you, or paddling alongside. They amplify the problem narrative many people bring to our work. We urge you to explore the other side of the story. The story of triumph, resilience, and constant change, despite the harshest of conditions. As Elliot Connie (2019) suggested, find the superhero in your client. We, the authors, have many stories of young clients surpassing others' expectations, emerging from a life of setbacks and routinely poor expectations to excel in their field.

We end this chapter with a family that demonstrated particular heroism. The mother referred her teenager who had been in and out of therapy since age six. The background story was troubling. The young 22-year-old mother bravely escaped ongoing domestic violence and sought family therapy to help with her clearly distressed young children. Citing "attachment therapy," the psychologist she sought support from instructed that when the children misbehave, evidenced through yelling or not sharing, she was to lock them in the basement, a room intentionally designed with only a small sleeping bag and water; a dungeon if you will. Sometimes overnight. The child's experience was disclosed to me (Will) during a canoeing expedition. Though familiar with the psychologist, we were uncertain whether this was true or not. The mother confirmed.

Upon returning home, we held a case conference with his school; his seventh school. With the young person's permission, we shared a quick version of his story and how us adults, volunteers in the helping professions, should provide a more supportive learning environment than he had ever experienced. He was expelled a week later for retaliating to a bully who had caused a significant injury. We tried the same at the next school, and the one after that. The problem behaviors his teachers reported were never witnessed during his outdoor therapy sessions. In fact, he became a mentor for first-time co-adventurers.

The mother called after a particularly bad day at school. Her son was crying over the phone saying he just wanted to move and go to a new school: the most prestigious boarding school in a neighboring country. "He would never be accepted," she said. We agreed. The current principal agreed and did not think it worth even trying. Months passed and he continued attending weekly adventures. The school issue was never raised.

It turned out he was mailing postcards to the principal in New Zealand and sending weekly emails asking for an interview. My phone rang one morning. The international dialing code +64 indicated the call was from, you guessed it, New Zealand. "Hi. This is Principal Jackie." She was calling to inquire about the young man and what supports the school could consider when they accept his enrolment in just two weeks' time. The mother was calling on the other line. The calls were merged. "We are so impressed with your son," the principal said. "That kind of initiative is exactly what our school is after. We just want to make sure we can make this work for all involved." The mother could not afford the school. She worked full time as an administrative assistant and cleaned holiday homes on the weekends when her kids were at their respective sports. "That will not be a problem," the principal assured. The mother cried in gratitude.

Two weeks later, he boarded a plane and off he went. He graduated as captain of his rugby team and returned home where he worked in hospitality and construction while pursuing a degree in economics.

Practitioners choose how to think about those they serve. No other adult in his life asked what he wanted. He kept it secret because no one ever took his best hopes seriously. His preferred future was impossible to everyone but Principal Jackie, who believed in him. His mother never endured another meeting to hear how difficult her son was. The two are no longer in therapy, and she is preparing to marry, both her boys to walk her down the aisle.

We can play a large role in people's lives. Before your next session, or adventure, invite yourself to be surprised. Not only by people's capabilities, but by how much they have already proved to you. Think of them at their best. It will make a difference (Flückiger et al., 2009). Be curious about their future, no matter how out of this world it seems. If they make it only 10% of the way there, they are still moving in that direction. What practitioners do outside can facilitate experiences where our co-adventurers feel inspired to share and be their best selves, providing genuine and attainable real-time clues to construct a miraculous future.

References

Adams, J. F., Piercy, F. P., & Jurich, J. A. (1991). Effects of solution focused therapy's "formula first session task" on compliance and outcome in family therapy. *Journal of Marital and Family Therapy*, *17*(3), 277–290. https://psycnet.apa.org/doi/10.1111/j.1752-0606.1991.tb00895.x

Anderson, S. (2014, August 12). When wilderness boot camps take tough love too far. *The Atlantic*. Retrieved from www.theatlantic.com/health/archive/2014/08/when-wilderness-boot-camps-take-tough-love-too-far/375582/

Berg, I. K., & Dolan, Y. (2001). *Tales of solutions: A collection of hope-inspiring stories.* W. W. Norton & Co.

Bond, C., Woods, K., Humphrey, N., Symes, W., & Green, L. (2013). Practitioner review: The effectiveness of solution focused brief therapy with children and families: A systematic and critical evaluation of the literature from 1990–2010. *Journal of Child Psychology and Psychiatry, 54*(7), 707–723. https://doi.org/10.1111/jcpp.12058

Bowen, D. J., & Neill, J. T. (2013). A meta-analysis of adventure therapy outcomes and moderators. *The Open Psychology Journal, 6*, Article 28-53. https://doi.org/10.2174/1874350120130802001

Brown, J., Dreis, S., & Nace, D. K. (1999). What really makes a difference in psychotherapy outcome? Why does managed care want to know? In M. A. Hubble, B. L. Duncan, & S. D. Miller (Eds.), *The heart and soul of change: What works in therapy* (pp. 389–406). American Psychological Association. https://doi.org/10.1037/11132-012

Caldwell, B. E. (2015). *Saving psychotherapy: How therapists can bring the talking cure back from the brink.* Ben Caldwell Labs.

Clark, J. P., Marmol, L. M., Cooley, R., & Gathercoal, K. (2004). The effects of wilderness therapy on the clinical concerns (on Axes I, II, and IV) of troubled adolescents. *Journal of Experiential Education, 27*(2), 213–232. https://doi.org/10.1177%2F105382590402700207

Connie, E. (2019). The solution-focused lesson in the Marvel universe: No spoilers. Retrieved from https://elliottconnie.com/no-spoilers/

de Shazer, S. (1984). The death of resistance. *Family Process, 23*(1), 11–17. https://doi.org/10.1111/j.1545-5300.1984.00011.x

de Shazer, S., & Berg, I. K. (1997). What works? Remarks on research aspects of solution-focused brief therapy. *Journal of Family Therapy, 19*(2), 121–124. https://doi.org/10.1111/1467-6427.00043

de Shazer, S., Dolan, L., Korman, H., Trepper, T., McCollum, E., & Berg, I. K. (2012). *More than miracles: The state of the art of solution-focused brief therapy.* Routledge.

Dobud, W. (2020). *Experiences of adventure therapy: A narrative inquiry* [Doctoral Dissertation]. Charles Sturt University.

Dobud, W. W., & Cavanaugh, D. L. (2020). Future direction for outdoor therapies. In N. J. Harper & W. W. Dobud (Eds.), *Outdoor Therapies: An Introduction to Practices, Possibilities, and Critical Perspectives* (pp. 188–202). Routledge.

Dobud, W. W., & Harper, N. J. (2018). Of dodo birds and common factors: A scoping review of direct comparison trials in adventure therapy. *Complementary Therapies in Clinical Practice, 31*, 16–24. https://doi.org/10.1016/j.ctcp.2018.01.005

Duncan, B. L. (2014). *On becoming a better therapist: Evidence-based practice one client at a time.* American Psychological Association.

Duncan, B. L., Miller, S. D., & Sparks, J. A. (2011). *The heroic client: A revolutionary way to improve effectiveness through client-directed, outcome-informed therapy.* John Wiley & Sons.

Eads, R., & Yee Lee, M. (2019). Solution focused therapy for trauma survivors: A review of the outcome literature. *Journal of Solution Focused Practices, 3*(1), 1–10.

Fernandez, E., Woldgabreal, Y., Day, A., Pham, T., Gleich, B., & Aboujaoude, E. (2021). Live psychotherapy by video versus in-person: A meta-analysis of efficacy and its relationship to types and targets of treatment. *Clinical Psychology & Psychotherapy.* https://doi.org/10.1002/cpp.2594

Flückiger, C., Caspar, F., Holtforth, M. G., & Willutzki, U. (2009). Working with patients' strengths: A microprocess approach. *Psychotherapy Research, 19*(2), 213–223.

Frank, J. D., & Frank, J. B. (1991). *Persuasion and healing: A comparative study of psychotherapy.* JHU Press.

Gass, M. A., & Gillis, H. L. (1995). Focusing on the "solution" rather than the "problem": Empowering client change in adventure experiences. *Journal of Experiential Education, 18*(2), 63–69. https://doi.org/10.1177%2F105382599501800202

Gass, M. A., Gillis, H. L., & Russell, K. C. (2012). *Adventure therapy: Theory, research, and practice.* Routledge.

Gass, M. A., Gillis, H. L., & Russell, K. C. (2020). *Adventure therapy. Theory, research, and practice* (2nd ed.) Routledge.

Government Accountability Office (GAO). (2007). *Residential treatment programs: Concerns regarding abuse and death in certain programs troubled youth.* United States Government Accountability Office.

Harper, N. J. (2009). Future paradigm or false idol: A cautionary tale of evidence-based practice for adventure education and therapy. *Journal of Experiential Education, 33*(1), 38–55. https://doi.org/10.1177%2F105382591003300104

Harper, N. J., & Dobud, W. W. (Eds.) (2020). *Outdoor therapies: An introduction to practices, possibilities, and critical perspectives*. Routledge.

Harper, N. J., & Doherty, T. J. (2020). An introduction to outdoor therapies. In N. J. Harper & W. W. Dobud (Eds.), *Outdoor therapies: An introduction to practices, possibilities, and critical perspectives* (pp. 3–15). Routledge.

Harper, N. J., Rose, K., & Segal, D. (2019). *Nature-based therapy: A practitioner's guide to working outdoors with children, youth, and families*. New Society Publishers.

McKergow, M. (2016). SFBT 2.0: The next generation of solution-focused brief therapy has already arrived. *Journal of Solution-Focused Brief Therapy*, 2(2), 1–17.

Meichenbaum, D., & Lilienfeld, S. O. (2018). How to spot hype in the field of psychotherapy: A 19-item checklist. *Professional Psychology: Research and Practice*, 49(1), 22–30. https://doi.org/10.1037/pro0000172

Miller, S. D., Hubble, M. A., Chow, D. L., & Seidel, J. A. (2013). The outcome of psychotherapy: Yesterday, today, and tomorrow. *Psychotherapy*, 50(1), 88–97. https://doi.org/10.1037/a0031097

Miller, S. D., Wampold, B. E., & Varhely, K. (2008). Direct comparisons of treatment modalities for youth disorders: A meta-analysis. *Psychotherapy Research*, 18(1), 5–14. https://doi.org/10.1080/10503300701472131

Natynczuk, S. (2014). Solution-focused practice as a useful addition to the concept of adventure therapy. *InterAction*, 6(1), 23–36.

Natynczuk, S. (2021). Co-adventuring for change: A solution focused framework for 'unspoken' therapy outdoors. *Relational Youth and Child Care*, 34(4), 59–65.

Natynczuk, S., & Dobud, W. W. (2021). Leave no trace, willful unknowing, and implications from the ethics of sustainability for solution-focused practice outdoors. *Journal of Solution Focused Practices*, 5(2), 7.

Norton, C. L., Tucker, A., Russell, K. C., Bettmann, J. E., Gass, M. A., Gillis, H. L., & Behrens, E. (2014). Adventure therapy with youth. *Journal of Experiential Education*, 37(1), 46–59. https://doi.org/10.1177%2F1053825913518895

Nylund, D., & Corsiglia, V. (1994). Becoming solution-focused forced in brief therapy: Remembering something important we already knew. *Journal of Systemic Therapies*, 13(1), 5–12. https://doi.org/10.1521/jsyt.1994.13.1.5

Pringle, G., Dobud, W. W., & Harper, N. J. (2021). The next frontier: Wilderness therapy and the treatment of complex trauma. In E. Brymer, M. Rogerson, & J. Barton (Eds.), *Nature and health: Physical activity in nature* (pp. 191–207). Routledge.

Ratner, H., George, E., & Iveson, C. (2012). *Solution focused brief therapy: 100 key points and techniques*. Routledge.

Selekman, M. D. (2005). *Pathways to change: Brief therapy with difficult adolescents* (2nd ed.) Guilford Publishing.

Shennan, G. (2019). *Solution-focused practice: Effective communication to facilitate change* (2nd ed.) Red Globe Press.

Sparks, J., Duncan, B. L., & Miller, S. D. (2007). Common factors and the uncommon heroism of youth. *Psychotherapy in Australia, 13*(2), 34–43.

Thomas, F. N. (2007). Possible limitations, misunderstandings, and misuses of solution-focused brief therapy. In T. Nelson & F. N. Thomas (Eds.), *Handbook of solution-focused brief therapy: Clinical applications* (pp. 404–421). The Haworth Press.

Tucker, A. R., Smith, A., & Gass, M. A. (2014). How presenting problems and individual characteristics impact successful treatment outcomes in residential and wilderness treatment programs. *Residential Treatment for Children and Youth, 31*(2), 135–153. https://doi.org/10.1080/0886571X.2014.918446

Walsh, V., & Golins, G. (1976). *The exploration of the Outward Bound process.* Colorado Outward Bound School.

Wampold, B. E., & Imel, Z. E. (2015). *The great psychotherapy debate: The evidence for what makes psychotherapy work* (2nd ed.) Routledge.

Wampold, B. E., Imel, Z. E., Laska, K. M., Benish, S., Miller, S. D., Flückiger, C., Del Re, A. C., Baardseth, T. P., & Budge, S. (2010). Determining what works in the treatment of PTSD. *Clinical Psychology Review, 30*(8), 923–933. https://doi.org/10.1016/j.cpr.2010.06.005

Weakland, J., Fisch, R., Watzlawick, P., & Bodin, A. (1974). Brief therapy: Focused problem resolution. *Family Process, 13*(2), 141–168. https://doi.org/10.1111/j.1545-5300.1974.00141.x

Yarbrough, J. L., & Thompson, C. L. (2002). Using single-participant research to assess counseling approaches on children's off-task behavior. *Professional School Counseling, 5*(5), 308–314.

2

On Becoming an Evidence-Informed Practitioner

"The moment philosophy supposes it can find a final and comprehensive solution, it ceases to be inquiry and becomes either apologetics or propaganda."

John Dewey (1938, p. 42)

In presenting a solution-focused approach to working with people in the outdoors, we remain mindful about the potential for misinterpretation that this approach is seemingly more effective than the next. As in our mission statement, we are intent on presenting a model for therapeutic practice in the outdoors and insight into becoming an evidence-informed practitioner, and to be the best we can possibly be at what we do well. To do this, we begin with examining what facilitates an "evidence-informed" outdoor therapy practice based on the definitions from various professional associations. We then discuss what works in therapy, based on the available process-outcome literature, and explore some key findings to ensure our work is grounded in the best available evidence. Outdoor therapy approaches have been criticized, and often rightly so, for being too diverse and poorly articulated (Russell & Farnum, 2004). Simply because two studies use the term wilderness therapy does not mean those two studies are researching anything with similarity (Fernee & Gabrielsen, 2020). Outcome research has also faced criticism for a lack of academic rigor (Dobud et al., 2020), and for condoning harmful, unethical practice (Rosen, 2020). For this reason, we present the evidence informing our practice and ethical considerations. We consider this most important before engaging in any discussion about which practice framework to incorporate, whether it be solution-focused or cognitive-behavioral. You could, for instance, incorporate ACT, CBT, DBT, ET, WT, AT, BAT, NBT, or any other T you like in your outdoor therapy work!

When we examined the professional bodies which accredit and license helping professionals around the world, we found a key theme of practice being

DOI: 10.4324/9781003217558-3

informed by the best available evidence. For example, the American Psychological Association (APA, 2020) stated clinical psychology practice is "grounded in science" (n.p.). Across international contexts, social work associations described that decisions should be based on "empirically based knowledge" in the United States (NASW, 2021, n.p.) and "research evidence" in Australia (AASW, 2020, p. 30). At the risk of listing association after association, we hope to stress the point that those working in a helping relationship are required to inform their decision-making processes with some empirical knowledge.

We are going to lean on a lot of quantitative research here. Privileging our philosophical stance of social construction and pragmatism, we do not maintain one method of inquiry is any better or more rigorous than the next, as we have written in the past (Dobud, 2020). Each piece of research should be critiqued on its own merit. We acknowledge various ways of knowing and the impacts of colonization on Indigenous cultures (Mitten, 2020). We examine this research because these studies speak the language of funders and policymakers, and dominate misinformed narratives of psychotherapy.

We do like the APA's (2005) definition of evidence-based practice as the "integration of the best available evidence with clinical expertise in the context of patient characteristics, culture, and preferences" (p. 5). This definition does not prefer quantitative over qualitative research and takes into account culture and client preferences making it useful for our striving for decolonization and client-directed programming (Natynczuk & Dobud, 2021). While the APA is an international influence for how we think about psychotherapy, their definition does not urge practitioners to choose one way of working over the next. It does not say cognitive-behavioral therapy is the best treatment for anxiety, or motivational interviewing is the best practice for substance misuse. Besides informing our practice about how therapy works, we use our *clinical expertise* and tailor our work to people's *characteristics, culture,* and *preferences*. Thus, evidence-based practice is a *verb* – something practitioners do together with their clients. It is not a *noun* – a treatment practitioners pick out of a hat. Conversely, and not to add confusion to the reader, when we describe outdoor, adventure, or wilderness therapy "programs," we are referring to programs as the noun, the organization, not a verb. Our aim is never to program people, nor do we believe our work is capable of such a thing.

No matter your profession or theoretical orientation, it is important to ground your practice in the evidence about what facilitates change and positive experiences. In this chapter, we describe key findings about therapy outcomes.

While we do not expect every reader of this text to gain access behind the paywall of peer-reviewed literature or spend their days off diving deeply into process and outcome research, there are a few replicated and essential findings worthy of serious consideration. These include: 1) therapy works; 2) the Dodo Bird verdict; 3) the variance in practitioner effects; and 4) how we can only improve outcomes one person at a time.

Therapy (Indoors) Works

The effectiveness of talking therapies have been questioned for nearly a century (Wampold & Imel, 2015). Proponents of different theoretical orientations, such as behaviorists and psychoanalysts, have engaged in historical debates as to *how* therapy outcomes are elicited. Both argued their method was best for reaching the mountain top. The issue was, however, both summited successfully.

Outcome studies typically involve a pre- and post-program evaluation model. Like many medical trials, a group of clients are provided a psychological measure at the start of the intervention and then the same measure at the end. In wilderness therapy, this is the common approach (see DeMille et al., 2018).

To increase the rigor of outcome research, researchers incorporate control groups. Most commonly used is a no-treatment control group where half the research participants receive no therapy at all. For example, Herbet (1998) randomly assigned participants to three different research groups. Experimental Group A participated in an eight-day adventure therapy program and a subsequent three-day program three months later. Experimental Group B received only the eight-day adventure therapy program. Group C was a no-treatment control group: they did not receive any adventure therapy services. After completion of the eight-day adventure therapy program, Experimental Groups A and B "reported higher levels of self-esteem and a shift towards an internal locus of control" (n.p.) than those who did not receive any adventure therapy (Group C). Herbet's study is good to examine due to the three conditions. In essence, the study compared adventure therapy versus adventure therapy versus nothing; and adventure therapy won out. We should hope so. With tongue planted firmly in cheek, it is good to be better than nothing at all. Because there was no experimental group receiving a service *different* to adventure therapy, we can only support the hypothesis that some adventure therapy is better than no therapy at all for those involved.

After a number of evaluations are conducted, researchers compile the available data in what is called a meta-analysis. These meta-analyses can provide an overview of the effects of a particular intervention.

Smith and Glass (1977) conducted the very first meta-analysis of psychotherapy outcomes. Their review included 375 studies of psychotherapy and counseling. Their findings provided "convincing evidence of the efficacy of psychotherapy. On average, a typical therapy client is better off than 75% of untreated individuals" (p. 752). This was a historical finding. At this time, there were arguments psychotherapy was indeed not effective. Smith and Glass (1977) demonstrated otherwise. Those in experimental groups receiving therapy were found better off than those in the no-treatment control groups. The study confirmed the effect of psychotherapy and found the therapy outcomes on par or surpassing commonly used medical treatments such as ibuprofen for a headache, bypass surgery, and chemotherapy for breast cancer (Wampold, 2007). For those reporting psychological or emotional distress, receiving therapy of any kind was significantly better than doing nothing at all. Like Herbet's (1998) study, Smith and Glass (1977) also compared the various forms of therapy to each other. Included in their analysis were a range of behavioral therapies, such as behavioral modification, and non-behavioral therapies, like psychodynamic or transactional analysis. While the behaviorists and non-behaviorists have had at it for the better part of a century, Smith and Glass found "virtually no difference in effectiveness" (p. 752) between the range of included therapies. All the therapies worked similarly well.

Meta-analyses like Smith and Glass' (1977) have continued. Miller et al. (2013) reviewed the available outcome research and found numerous meta-analyses, across a range of models, to support and confirm something we have not heard enough of: Therapy works! What the researchers have struggled to answer is: *How and why does it work?* This brings us to the verdict of a very clever Dodo Bird.

Dodo Bird Verdict

For years, Will's refrigerator holds a magnet of a dodo bird from the Oxford University Museum of Natural History. I (Stephan) mailed it to him from England in 2018 after he published a paper alongside our good friend and colleague Nevin Harper from Canada. The paper was titled: "Of dodo birds and common factors: A scoping review of direct comparison trials in adventure therapy" (Dobud & Harper, 2018).

The following excerpt comes from the Dodo paper:

> In 1936, friend and classmate of B. F. Skinner, psychologist Saul Rosenzweig, published *Some Implicit Common Factors in Diverse Methods of Psychotherapy*, in which he cited Lewis Carroll's *Alice's Adventures in Wonderland*. In Carroll's story, Alice's tears had drenched the animals and a race was held for the animals to dry themselves. At the end, the Dodo bird was asked who had won, and he declared, "*Everybody* has won, and *all* must have prizes" [p. 412, emphasis in original]. In his short paper, Rosenzweig asked, if all the different models of therapy were equally effective for a diverse range of clients, then was each model of psychotherapy a winner as well?
>
> (Harper & Dobud, 2018, p. 16)

Rosenzweig (1936) was 41 years ahead of Smith and Glass (1977). Therapy worked and all the modalities deserved prizes. What Dobud and Harper (2018) explored was whether this finding relates to therapy outdoors. They conducted a literature search to find every time therapy was taken outside compared to participation in another type of therapy omitting outdoor or adventurous conditions. While some researchers will compare participation with no-treatment controls, they were interested in direct comparison trials. Instead of no-treatment control groups, the studies included conditions where all research participants received some form of an established therapy. The findings supported the Dodo Bird's verdict. Of the 13 studies, all but two found a familiar conclusion: No differences in outcomes between the different modes of therapy. This required further examination. Is it possible those two studies can debunk the Dodo Bird's exclamation from nearly 100 years ago?

Tucker et al.'s (2013) study was large and robust. It included a sample of 1,113 young people in Ohio who received either adventure therapy, adventure therapy with psychological counseling, psychological counseling, or psychological and group counseling in a community mental health setting. There were two aspects of this study leading to the conclusion of more research being needed. The first related to the very nature of the various experimental groups. There were 18 participants who received adventure therapy alone. 104 received adventure therapy and psychological counseling. 53 received psychological counseling and group therapy, and the remaining 652 participants received psychological counseling only. These are unequal experimental groups and, typical in outcome studies, the larger the group the smaller the effect. In this case, we could not state the outcomes of 18 participants, only 50% of which achieved clinically reliable change, reflected a more efficacious treatment than 652 (42.5% of which showed reliable change). The second related to the outcome measures.

Based on the problem severity scale used by the researchers, it was clear the participants receiving only adventure therapy were experiencing higher levels of distress than the other experimental groups. For Brown et al. (1999), high levels of distress are a great predictor of larger effect sizes on statistical measures. It is hard to make the claim there was enough to suggest it was adventure therapy alone that led to the study outcomes.

The second study had a similar finding, though it was the other way around! Magle-Haberek et al. (2012) found residential treatment outperformed wilderness therapy, now referred to as outdoor behavioral healthcare (OBH) in the United States. Like the previous study though, those receiving residential treatment were, on average, reporting higher levels of distress at the start of treatment. In this case, we could not suggest indoor residential treatment was more effective for adolescents than outdoor wilderness therapy. What is missing in order to claim outdoor therapy has active specific ingredients are equivalent experimental groups where half participants reporting similar levels of distress receive an outdoor therapy and the others receive a bonafide indoor psychotherapy.

Achieving high-standard, randomized clinical trials in outdoor therapy is hard. Norwegian outdoor therapy researchers Gabrielsen et al. (2015) did not succeed in reaching this so-called "gold-standard" of research. Research participants need to agree to take part in any trial. They sign an informed consent document and agree to the parameters set out by the researchers. Adolescents referred to the hospital at which this team was employed were informed about the trial. Should they wish to participate, they would receive either high-quality traditional outpatient talk therapy sessions or the hospital's new and innovative wilderness therapy program. The young people preferred the latter. Those randomized to the treatment-as-usual group were not happy. One told the researchers it felt like Santa had brought them a present, only to take it away again. They preferred the great outdoors. The research team honored the clients' preferences and the trial was abandoned. We assume ongoing pursuits for clinical trials will end similarly.

At this stage, we find it necessary to hit the pause button and revisit our argument. We began this chapter stressing the importance of informing outdoor therapy practice based on the best available evidence. We began by zooming out and asking the question, *Does therapy work?* We do not think twice about our answer. Psychotherapy outcomes are robust (Miller et al., 2013). The second question, *How does therapy work?* is harder to answer. Many advocates for incorporating the outdoors in their therapy practice may argue it is the adventure, such as climbing a rock wall, or simply the time in nature that leads to improved wellbeing. However, when we look at the Dodo Bird's verdict, these components did not outperform the types of therapy not including those factors. In this case, it is hard to say assertively what specific ingredients are required to effectively take therapeutic practice outdoors.

The argument growing in this chapter is one that has existed since the dawn of psychotherapy research (Wampold & Imel, 2015). On one side are proponents who believe therapy works like medicine. They argue therapeutic change occurs because of the specific ingredients of taking therapy outdoors. While we have found most outdoor therapy practitioners push back at the idea of using therapy and medicine in the same sentence, outcome research focusing on one type of nature-based service and removing the therapist from the discussion undermines the therapy altogether. On the other side, where we find ourselves firmly positioned, is that change is entirely contextual and constructed between practitioners and active participants.

If the Dodo's verdict holds up, a future research agenda should shy away from focusing on the model itself. What if instead of empirically supported therapies, we had empirically supported therapists? If evidence-based practice is a verb – something practitioners do – then we need to explore if there are any pantheoretical actions practitioners take that lead to improved outcomes. Additionally, are there routine shortcomings we can glean from the evidence? We strengthen this argument by looking at therapist or practitioner effects and provide implications for outdoor therapy practice.

Practitioner Effects

Each practitioner has their strengths. Some are funny, others deeply insightful. Some better at group work and others more effective one to one. If you are reading this, you are probably already working therapeutically in the outdoors or seriously considering taking the next step to do so. Remember at the start of this chapter we argued many professional bodies claim helping professionals should ground their practice based on the best evidence as to how therapy works. Since then we solidified the effectiveness of therapy and used the available literature to suggest it is not the type of therapy provided that is largely responsible for therapeutic outcomes, nor is it the setting. If it is not likely the type of therapy, there must be a different factor to consider.

Wampold and Brown (2005) conducted a large-scale study of 581 clinicians who worked with over 6,000 clients. The researchers examined a range of factors to predict what led to client change, including how effective the practitioners were on average. Of the client factors, age, gender, and diagnosis made no difference to outcomes. For the practitioners, years of experience, training, or the theoretical orientation also made no difference. What the authors found was enlightening. The clients who saw the best, most effective therapists had at least 50% better outcomes and dropped out at rates more than 50% below those who worked with "average" practitioners. Average might be a troubling word, but let us remember on (mean) average, therapy works and works really well! That said, here lies the problem with assuming specific therapy models, such as cognitive-behavioral or motivational interviewing, are responsible for client change. No matter how tightly we control our outdoor therapy model, whether through ongoing training, supervision, or even manualizing service delivery, some practitioners routinely elicit better outcomes than others.

Here is something we all know, but seldom discuss. Two practitioners, working for the same agency, delivering the same service to a similar set of clients, are likely to elicit two totally different sets of outcomes. If larger agencies measured individual practitioner outcomes, they would likely find a bell curve based on their practitioners' performance. Lots would be average (95% between −2 and +2 standard deviations of the mean), a few well below average, and a few high-level performers. Baldwin et al. (2007) found 97% of the difference between therapist outcomes is in their ability to form stronger therapeutic relationships!

The outdoor therapies are eclectic, diverse, and include a range of models from adventure therapy to wilderness therapy to nature-based therapy (Harper & Dobud, 2020). Despite the evidence making it clear models are only responsible for the smallest amount of variance in client change, Wampold and Imel (2015) found in their review of outcome data that practitioners who do not align with a particular therapeutic model can wander aimlessly in their practice. Models provide us with a theoretical framework and a practical rationale for our work with clients.

While Carl Rogers' (1957) core conditions of change are key to any effective therapy, they are not enough. Some clinical trials compare bona-fide empirically supported therapies to what has been referred to as "relational counseling." This is an experimental condition containing all the ingredients of normal talk therapy – a therapist, a client, a relationship, a couch, a room, you get the point – but there is no model. The client does not know they are receiving a therapy with no psychological rationale or ritual, but the therapist does. It does not work as well (Wampold & Imel, 2015). The therapeutic alliance consists of more than just a relational bond. It includes agreement of the purpose of our work and the methods, rituals, and techniques that will help to achieve that purpose. Outdoor therapy practitioners require a theoretical framework to inform their practice. Taking solution-focused brief therapy outdoors is simply one way to go about this, especially as it is supported by a practical leadership model and a strong person-centered ethic.

Another question, quite relevant to outdoor therapies, is what training and qualifications are required to deliver such services. In the United States, adventure therapy is often defined as a service provided by mental health professionals (Gass et al., 2012), while Australian and many European contexts may not require such clinical education or qualification. Participants of outdoor therapy often interact with various professionals with no clinical training. For instance, a wilderness therapy expedition may be led by outdoor guides and one clinical psychotherapist. For this reason, our book is designed to be useful for the experienced clinician and the outdoor professionals who are effective and essential to working therapeutically outdoors. We do not engage in debates about what is or is not "therapy," nor who is most qualified to deliver effective services, in this context.

In some instances it seems being a professional counselor gives little advantage. Karlsruher (1974) and Durlak (1979) found non-professionals tended to be more effective than professional counselors. Hattie et al. (1984) found what they referred to as "paraprofessionals" as being more effective than trained therapists in long-term counseling (>12 weeks). Berman and Norton (1985) found no overall differences between the two. Strupp and Hadley (1979) found non-professionals just as helpful as professionals. It seems personal qualities and interpersonal skills are most helpful for getting useful outcomes. Non-professional counselors tended to be more authentic, less likely to apply labels to clients, to provide safety, and clients attributed success to themselves rather than to the expertise of the therapist. Difficult cases tended to be referred on and there were limited case-loads. Those without clinical training tended to be highly motivated to help, more likely to be culturally compatible, and gave more time to clients.

Importantly and based on the available evidence, we do not argue university training and specific qualifications make for a more effective practitioner, though we are employed by such institutions and highly recommend the pursuit of lifelong learning. If you are interested in ongoing education, choose your discipline based on finances and what sparks your interest (Caldwell, 2015). Focusing on *your* model of service delivery and using the best available evidence to inform your practice is key. Similarly, it is vital to revisit the ethics of your work.

People have worked therapeutically in the outdoors for decades and the evidence supports such approaches (Bowen & Neill, 2013). We cannot rely on our model of therapy or theoretical stance, whether indoors or out, solution-focused or trauma-informed, to do this work for us. Models do not work in isolation from the context of who we are as practitioners, the person we tailor our work towards, and the relationship we construct together. While it is clear all models rely on a strong therapeutic relationship, we use the following section to present the outcome literature as to why we must adopt a *relationship-focused* stance above and beyond our focus on the models and techniques we use.

Therapeutic Alliance

Terms like the therapeutic relationship, working alliance, and therapeutic alliance are often used interchangeably. However, Norcross and Lambert (2011) described the therapeutic relationship as incredibly broad, within which is the more easily defined therapeutic alliance. The alliance is one of the most evidence-based factors for predicting outcomes. Bordin (1979) provided what would become a settled upon definition of the alliance to include a relational bond, consensus about the aims or purpose of therapy, and agreement about what the practitioner and client will do together. That agreement should include some expectation that what the practitioner does is likely to help. This does not mean the practitioner is responsible for the change necessarily; more that a client's rating of the therapeutic alliance is a reliable factor for predicting outcomes. This is why along with outcomes, it is important to inquire about the client's perception of the alliance; to establish a relationship where co-adventurers can let us know when something is missing. If we do not seek this feedback, it is unlikely we will be able to adjust our approach in time. Additionally, if we become defensive when we receive negative feedback, we communicate we are not taking clients' experience in therapy seriously. This can lead to a damning power imbalance and rupture the quality of the therapeutic relationship.

Over 1,100 separate studies support the impact of the therapeutic alliance on outcomes (Norcross & Lambert, 2011), making the alliance one of the most research-supported factors in describing how therapy works; the alliance impacts outcomes five to nine times more than the specific model being delivered. To put this in perspective, funding bodies and third party payers, such as the Medicare system in Australia, often fund practitioners based on the type of therapy they deliver, in this case cognitive-behavioral therapy

(Miller et al., 2013). Those decisions are based on anything but the available research. Consider the argument we presented in Chapter 1. Why are third party payers privileging the counseling room over telehealth or the outdoors? Of immense importance to us is the quality of the working alliance, and this has led to us championing the idea of co-adventuring for change.

Most important here is the client's rating of the alliance, not the practitioner's. Consider empathy, one of Roger's (1957) core conditions of change. When we return from an outdoor therapy session, we do not walk in the door and when asked about the day proclaim, "You should have seen how empathetic I was!" That is, of course, ridiculous. It is our clients who, ideally, go home to their partners, friends, or colleagues and say, "My therapist was really tuned in with me today!" It is the client's perception of the therapy that predicts outcomes, not the practitioner's.

The variance between certain practitioners often materializes in their clients' ratings of the therapeutic alliance. Said another way, some practitioners simply tend to engage a more diverse range of clients. Eliciting this engagement, often through a strong therapeutic alliance, could be the factor differentiating the best from the rest (Baldwin et al., 2007).

We are passionate advocates for opening the therapy room door and engaging in therapy outdoors. We would love to see more people do it! Simply taking a client outside does not guarantee your effectiveness. There is too much context: the person of the client, your average effectiveness, your ability to engage certain people, and a myriad of other factors. Similarly, the research suggests that while engaging with a certain person, practitioners may not be the best person to know if they are on track, off track, or if there has been a rupture in the therapeutic alliance. There will also be moments we need to partner with those we work with to head in a different direction. This is a problem for practitioners from all disciplines. What we do might not work for all clients. The real opportunity for growth and improving a person's experience of care is to determine when we are effective, and more importantly, when we are not. Then we can do something about it before it is too late.

Therapeutic Alliance Outdoors

While outdoors, it is not unusual for everyone to spend hours in close proximity, helping each other with tasks, safety, navigation, and so on. Teamwork, mutual dependence, and common endeavors remain strong themes. Aspects of our personal lives and personality are difficult to keep hidden when spending so much time together. This picture of close cooperation in an endeavor starkly contrasts with a traditional therapy setting indoors, or even a therapeutic hour outside where talking is the main therapy. On expeditions, there are many opportunities for participants to learn of their guides' or instructors' likes, dislikes, fears, phobias, habits, hobbies, abilities, biases, humor, nearest and dearest, and so forth. Boundaries can be tested much more readily. Personal questions can be difficult to avoid. Altogether the therapeutic alliance can be tested to destruction on many occasions. I (Stephan) have witnessed this with an aspirant guide who, thinking it helpful, told a client about a personal experience only to have information used against them in a hurtful and public verbal attack. Likewise physical boundaries have to be respected, for example, always having a witness when adjusting harnesses. There are tricky grey areas, such as working with children with additional needs wanting to hold hands, and possibly times when personal care becomes part of the job. Context is such an important consideration. It is always best to have another adult as a witness, and to think through these additional roles with referrers and colleagues well before they become an issue, and to establish a code of conduct informed by child protection best practice in your cultural context.

Outdoor therapy providers have a challenge in balancing the role of therapist and outdoor leader. Anything less than authenticity, honesty, and competence can expose a leader as not up to the job and ruin any kind of quality relationship, let alone one as special as a therapeutic alliance. Equally, there are plenty of opportunities to foster collaboration, honest communication, respect, and trust, which help build a robust and transparent relationship and within "professional boundaries." In Chapter 4, we talk about a leadership framework consistent with our therapeutic model. Foremost in our thinking is ensuring leadership fits with therapy, and that every aspect of our therapy is efficiently aligned.

We remain cautious in telling people what kind of relationships to establish when working therapeutically outdoors. Any specific idea or technique risks becoming prey to the Dodo Bird. Our advice on relationship building will typically be no more impactful than what you already know. Still, there are clues we have learned from our work and research endeavors. These include the establishing of *real relationships*, the participant *feeling valued*, and avoiding becoming *solution-forced*, which we explore throughout subsequent chapters (Dobud, 2020).

A recent meta-analysis by Gelso et al. (2018) explored how real relationships impact psychotherapy outcomes. The authors defined the real relationship as:

> the personal relationship between patient and therapist marked by the extent to which it is genuine with the other and perceives/experiences the other in ways that are realistic. The strength of the real relationship is determined by both the extent to which it exists and the degree to which it is positive and favourable.
>
> (p. 434)

Qualitative research into outdoor therapy relationships reinforced this statement (Dobud, 2020). Allow space for informal conversations, both between practitioner and participant, but also among co-adventurers when conducting group or expedition-based work (Mitten, 1994). While practitioners cannot abolish the power differential, consider how you can be as "down in the dirt" as you can with your co-adventurers, as one past outdoor therapy participant put it. Some practitioners may hold values against sharing personal information, there is certainly a line to be drawn on how much is shared. Practitioners can seek supervision and discuss how to best respond when asked these types of questions. Leaving a client's question unanswered can drive a wedge between the two of you, so practice care, tact, and diplomacy.

Outdoor therapy endeavors require careful planning. During a camping trip, practitioners may be required to organize food, prepare activities like rock climbing, and schedule for each day. Hold on to your itinerary loosely. Focus on your co-adventurer's experience and preferences. Their view of the alliance, which includes your relational bond *and* the work itself, requires most of our attention. If we hold onto our models and scheduling too firmly, we risk becoming solution-*forced*. If a co-adventurer prefers some small changes, we do not label them as resistant or difficult. We avoid over theorizing why they are not responding to our expertise, instead focusing on delivering a more useful and engaging experience. It is their adventure; their therapy.

Improving Outcomes One Person at a Time

Part III of this book dives deeper into this topic of outcome monitoring and seeking client feedback. While most practitioners contend they do elicit client feedback, many do not systematically, and more importantly routinely. We view this as not only essential to becoming evidence-informed, it is also an ethical consideration.

Of course, not everyone benefits from therapy. Lambert and Ogles (2009) reported 30–50% of participants experience no change, or even worse, deteriorate while in our care. The literature and evidence tells us practitioners are not very good at identifying who is at risk of dropping out or who is getting worse in our care. For example, Hannan et al. (2005) found practitioners were rarely able to predict who on their caseload experienced a deterioration of their wellbeing. They urged practitioners to incorporate outcome measures into their work in order to build evidence, in real time, as to who was not experiencing change.

We find Caldwell's (2015) metaphor of getting into a taxi blindfolded useful here. Clients arrive motivated by something. Similarly, people get in a taxi because they want to get somewhere. Now imagine getting in a taxi blindfolded. You tell the driver where you want to go. However, while blindfolded, you cannot follow the route the driver is taking you, whether they are running red lights, or how expensive the fare is. Similarly, you are unaware if the driver has previously driven someone like you effectively and safely.

We have systematically and routinely collected client feedback for more than a decade. We want to be the best we can be for our clients. The pre-/post-program evaluations we described before have inherent limitations. For example, if a client is not progressing, practitioners may overlook this until after the program when the outcome measure is re-administered.

It was the pioneering work of Kenneth I. Howard et al. (1986, 1993, 1996) which really championed *dose effect* in psychotherapy, an area we know little about in nature-based therapies (Harper et al., 2019). Borrowing this term from medicine, Howard et al. (1986) began researching *how much* therapy is required to elicit change. After all, there are various constructs about time in therapy. Take solution-focused *brief* therapy, for example. We question the relevance of constructs of brief versus long term. Practitioners should strive towards a person's desired future as efficiently and quickly as possible, immediately working towards a time when the therapy is not needed. Still, there is an important lesson to be learned from Howard and colleagues' dose-effect research. What made Howard et al.' (1986, 1993, 1996) work so important was building the evidence of when change is likely to occur, no matter a practitioner's theoretical stance. The evidence is clear that the longer we work with someone not experiencing any desired benefit, the less likely they are to at all! We should look out for early change, and if it is not experienced, seriously consider adjusting the therapy or referring them to another practitioner. Roughly 30% of people demonstrate improvement by the second session, 60–65% by the seventh session, 70–75% within six months, and 85%

after one year. If a client is not reporting progress early on, change becomes less and less likely.

Emerging from the dose-effect literature is another framework for interpreting change and the length of certain interventions: *the good-enough level*, which is a useful aspect of the solution-focused approach (Shennan, 2019). Where Howard et al. (1986) presented the statistics on how quickly change should occur for the average therapy recipient, Falkenström et al. (2016) described the good-enough-level involved practitioners deciding with participants on when to conclude their work together based on a satisfactory outcome. Our relationships might be brief for those who respond quickly and longer for those whose trajectory of change is more akin to a light stroll up a hill. Still, it is vital we are evaluating each client's progress systematically and routinely.

How we monitor client progress is examined further in Chapter 9. At this point it is worth providing a brief description of what this looks like in the outdoors. Upon first meeting a potential client, we explain we like to measure progress in therapy and really benefit from them letting us know where they are now so we can make sure we are on the right track. We then provide the simple and ultra-brief Outcome Rating Scale (Miller et al., 2003) which the client fills out.

With practice, this is achieved in less than a minute. The measure is administered each and every session. Different considerations are taken during expeditions and in residential treatment. At the end of the session, we communicate being interested in examining how it felt to take part in the session. We provide, again, an ultra-brief scale; the Session Rating Scale (Duncan et al., 2003). The client completes the scale and we attempt to elicit any negative feedback helping us to improve for the next session. It is likely anyone "complaining" is invested in your service and wants things to be better, and as top companies invest in knowing the *voice of the customer*, it is easily apparent that improving customer experiences and their satisfaction is important (Kotler & Keller, 2009).

Like solution-focused practice, this process is deceptively simple. Measuring outcomes alone will not improve our efficacy. Just like all therapeutic approaches, there is an art to eliciting client feedback. After all, as practitioners we sit in a privileged position, making it harder to receive negative feedback. Duncan et al. (2007), for example, found "the disparity in power between therapist and client, combined with socioeconomic, ethic, or racial differences, can make it difficult for our clients to tell us we're on the wrong track" (p. 42). The authors described imagining what it would be like to see a lawyer, dentist, or doctor if you believed they were not acting in your best interest. You would leave and not go back. Or worse, you could stay and not receive your desired outcome!

Routine outcome monitoring helps in a number of ways. First, it provides a framework for practitioners to briefly, easily, and robustly measure their outcomes. If we know our baseline effectiveness, we can know where we need to improve; like a golfer and their par. Second, by monitoring outcomes each session we are alerted to the people in our care who are not improving or feeling as though we are leading them in an ill-favored direction. Third, these practices can help us to leave our biases at the door. We do not know what is best for each person until we ask and we cannot know if we are headed towards their preferred future if we do not inquire. Measuring outcomes and eliciting feedback provides a tool for catching the people who fall through the cracks. We use this framework to engage the disengaged and demonstrate that even though we may ask those we work with to be vulnerable with us, we too are walking the walk. We put ourselves out there each session or every day of a grueling expedition. This helps us be at our best, one person at a time and one session or one day at a time. Outcome monitoring and feedback helps us to be sure we are primarily working towards our client's own best interests.

Vanity Metrics

You will notice in this discussion of how therapy works that we did not talk about the impact of natural settings on outdoor therapy outcomes. After all, most of us interested in outdoor therapy come to this work based on our own adventures and outdoor experiences. Wanting to give something back is a commonly heard reason for choosing an adventure-based career. However, when we talk about outcomes in relation to those we serve, the co-adventurers, practitioners should avoid getting bogged down in vanity metrics (Chow, 2018). We get stuck when measuring what we think is most important, such as asking clients to report how important time in nature is. When practitioners and advocates for certain modalities measure what they find most important, they silence the voice of the minority, in this case the clients. What would change if we only measured what clients want? We should focus our outcomes on precisely what brings people to therapy and factors which contribute significantly to client progress, such as a strong therapeutic alliance.

Funding bodies contract many outdoor therapy providers by asking them to measure what the funding body values – typically "butts in seats" or how many programs you have rolled out in your community. Of course, they want their money to reach as many people as possible, though this tends to discount what the recipients of these programs value. We encourage practitioners, as recommended by Chow (2018), to measure what matters to your clients. Measuring anything else might make you look good, but these areas of focus are unlikely to make a difference to the people asking for help.

Conclusion

The research informing our work is often dry, dense, and full of language sounding not too relevant to everyday work outdoors. We hope that this compact illustration of what works in therapy provides an actual grounding to what you already do. Some might be experienced outdoor therapy providers and others considering this work, or wondering how to enter the field. We hope the Dodo Bird's verdict gives you no pause. Therapy outdoors should no longer be considered an "alternative" since our outcomes are on par with everything else, even those highly researched therapies like CBT, as Stigsdotter et al. (2018) found. That should be encouraging.

Who delivers the service is a much bigger determinant of outcome than the type of service being provided. We cannot rely on the outdoors to do this work for us or for the specific questions we ask to operate void of personal and interpersonal context. Becoming evidence-informed means we acknowledge it takes work and a certain mindset to tailor our approaches to each person who comes through the door, or enters the canoe or cave with us. We are not in the position to determine what is working in another's life. If we guess wrong, we may not see them again, or worse, do harm. It is their perspective of our work which must be privileged above all else.

References

American Psychological Association [APA]. (2005). *Report of the 2005 Presidential Task for on Evidence-Based Practice.* American Psychological Association. Retrieved from www.apa.org/practice/resources/evidence/evidence-based-report.pdf

American Psychological Association [APA]. (2020). *About APA.* American Psychological Association. Retrieved June 12, 2020 from www.apa.org/about/

Australian Association of Social Workers [AASW]. (2020). *Code of ethics.* Australian Association of Social Workers. www.aasw.asn.au/document/item/13400

Baldwin, S. A., Wampold, B. E., & Imel, Z. E. (2007). Untangling the alliance-outcome correlation: Exploring the relative importance of therapist and patient variability in the alliance. *Journal of Consulting and Clinical Psychology*, 75(6), 842–852. https://psycnet.apa.org/doi/10.1037/0022-006X.75.6.842

Berman, J. S., & Norton, N. C. (1985). Does professional training make a therapist more effective? *Psychological Bulletin*, 98(2), 401–407. https://doi.org/10.1037/0033-2909.98.2.401

Bordin, E. S. (1979). The generalizability of the psychoanalytic concept of the working alliance. *Psychotherapy: Theory, research & practice*, 16(3), 1–9.

Bowen, D. J., & Neill, J. T. (2013). A meta-analysis of adventure therapy outcomes and moderators. *The Open Psychology Journal*, 6, Article 28-53. https://doi.org/10.2174/1874350120130802001

Brown, J., Dreis, S., & Nace, D. K. (1999). What really makes a difference in psychotherapy outcome? Why does managed care want to know? In M. A. Hubble, B. L. Duncan, & S. D. Miller (Eds.), *The heart and soul of change: What works in therapy* (pp. 389–406). American Psychological Association. https://doi.org/10.1037/11132-012

Caldwell, B. E. (2015). *Saving psychotherapy: How therapists can bring the talking cure back from the brink*. Ben Caldwell Labs.

Chow, D. L. (2018). Vanity metrics: Do we value what we measure, or measure what we value? *Frontiers of Psychotherapist Development*. Retrieved from https://darylchow.com/frontiers/vanity-metrics-do-we-value-what-we-measure-or-do-measure-what-we-value/

DeMille, S., Tucker, A. R., Gass, M. A., Javorski, S., VanKanegan, C., Talbot, B., & Karoff, M. (2018). The effectiveness of outdoor behavioral healthcare with struggling adolescents: A comparison group study a contribution for the special issue: Social innovation in child and youth services. *Children and Youth Services Review*, 88, 241–248. https://doi.org/10.1016/j.childyouth.2018.03.015

Dewey, J. (1938). *Logic: The theory of inquiry*. Holt, Rinehart and Winston.

Dobud, W. W. (2020). *Experiences of adventure therapy: A narrative inquiry* [Doctoral Dissertation]. Charles Sturt University.

Dobud, W. W., Cavanaugh, D. L., & Harper, N. J. (2020). Adventure therapy and routine outcome monitoring of treatment: The time is now. *Journal of Experiential Education*, 43(3), 262–276. https://doi.org/10.1177%2F1053825920911958

Dobud, W. W., & Harper, N. J. (2018). Of dodo birds and common factors: A scoping review of direct comparison trials in adventure therapy. *Complementary Therapies in Clinical Practice*, 31, 16–24. https://doi.org/10.1016/j.ctcp.2018.01.005

Duncan, B. L., Miller, S., & Hubble, M. (2007). How being bad can make you better. *Psychotherapy Networker, 31*(5), 36–46.

Duncan, B. L., Miller, S. D., Sparks, J. A., Claud, D. A., Reynolds, L. R., Brown, J., & Johnson, L. D. (2003). The Session Rating Scale: Preliminary psychometric properties of a "working" alliance measure. *Journal of Brief Therapy, 3*(1), 3–12.

Falkenström, F., Josefsson, A., Berggren, T., & Holmqvist, R. (2016). How much therapy is enough? Comparing dose-effect and good-enough models in two different settings. *Psychotherapy, 53*(1), 130–139. https://doi.org/10.1037/pst0000039

Fernee, C. R., & Gabrielsen, L. E. (2020). Wilderness therapy. In N. J. Harper & W. W. Dobud (Eds.) *Outdoor therapies: An introduction to practices, possibilities, and critical perspectives* (pp. 69–80). Routledge.

Gabrielsen, L. E., Fernee, C. R., Aasen, G. O., & Eskedal, L. T. (2015). Why randomized trials are challenging within adventure therapy research: Lessons learned in Norway. *Journal of Experiential Education, 39*(1), 5–14. https://doi.org/10.1177%2F1053825915607535

Gass, M. A., Gillis, H. L., & Russell, K. C. (2012). *Adventure therapy: Theory, research, and practice.* Routledge.

Gelso, C. J., Kivlighan, D. M., Jr., & Markin, R. D. (2018). The real relationship and its role in psychotherapy outcome: A meta-analysis. *Psychotherapy, 55*(4), 434–444. https://doi.org/10.1037/pst0000183

Hannan, C., Lambert, M. J., Harmon, C., Nielsen, S. L., Smart, D. W., Shimokawa, K., et al. (2005). A lab test and algorithms for identifying clients at risk for treatment failure. *Journal of Clinical Psychology: In Session, 61*, 155–163. https://doi.org/10.1002/jclp.20108

Harper, N. J., & Dobud, W. W. (Eds.) (2020). *Outdoor Therapies: an introduction to practices, possibilities, and critical perspectives.* Routledge.

Harper, N. J., Rose, K., & Segal, D. (2019). *Nature-based therapy: A practitioner's guide to working outdoors with children, youth, and families.* New Society Publishers.

Hattie, J. A., Sharpley, C. F., & Rogers, H. J. (1984). Comparative effectiveness of professional and paraprofessional helpers. *Psychological Bulletin, 95*(3), 534–541.

Herbet, J. T. (1998). Therapeutic effects of participating in an adventure therapy program. *Rehabilitation Counseling Bulletin, 41*(3), 201–216.

Howard, K. I., Kopta, S. M., Krause, M. S., & Orlinsky, D. E. (1986). The dose–effect relationship in psychotherapy. *American Psychologist, 41*(2), 159–164. https://doi.org/10.1037/0003-066X.41.2.159

Howard, K. I., Lueger, R. J., Maling, M. S., & Martinovich, Z. (1993). A phase model of psychotherapy outcome: Causal mediation of change. *Journal of Consulting and Clinical Psychology, 61*(4), 678–685. https://doi.org/10.1037/0022-006X.61.4.678

Howard, K. I., Moras, K., Brill, P. L., Martinovich, Z., & Lutz, W. (1996). Evaluation of psychotherapy: Efficacy, effectiveness, and patient progress. *American Psychologist*, 51(10), 1059–1064. https://doi.org/10.1037/0003-066X.51.10.1059

Karlsruher, A. E. (1974). The nonprofessional as a psychotherapeutic agent: A review of the empirical evidence pertaining to his effectiveness. *American Journal of Community Psychology*, 2(1), 61–77. https://doi.org/10.1007/BF00894155

Kotler, P., & Keller, K. L. (2009). *Marketing management* (13th ed.) Pearson Education Ltd.

Lambert, M. J., & Ogles, B. M. (2009). Using clinical significance in psychotherapy outcome research: The need for a common procedure and validity data. *Psychotherapy Research*, 19(4–5), 493–501. https://doi.org/10.1080/10503300902849483

Magle-Haberek, N. A., Tucker, A. R., & Gass, M. A. (2012). Effects of program differences with wilderness therapy and Residential Treatment Center (RTC) programs. *Residential Treatment for Children & Youth*, 29(3), 202–218. https://doi.org/10.1080/0886571X.2012.697433

Miller, S. D., Duncan, B. L., Brown, J., Sparks, J. A., & Claud, D. A. (2003). The outcome rating scale: A preliminary study of the reliability, validity, and feasibility of a brief visual analog measure. *Journal of Brief Therapy*, 2(2), 91–100.

Miller, S. D., Hubble, M. A., Chow, D. L., & Seidel, J. A. (2013). The outcome of psychotherapy: Yesterday, today, and tomorrow. *Psychotherapy*, 50(1), 88–97. https://doi.org/10.1037/a0031097

Mitten, D. (1994). Ethical considerations in adventure therapy: A feminist critique. *Women & Therapy*, 15(3–4), 55–84. https://doi.org/10.1300/J015v15n03_06

Mitten, D. (2020). Critical perspectives on outdoor therapy practices. In N. J. Harper & W. W. Dobud (Eds.). *Outdoor therapies: An introduction to practices, possibilities, and critical perspectives* (pp. 175–187). Routledge.

National Association of Social Workers [NASW]. (2021). Read the code of ethics. National Association of Social Workers. Retrieved June 12, 2021 from www.socialworkers.org/About/Ethics/Code-of-Ethics/Code-of-Ethics-English

Natynczuk, S., & Dobud, W. W. (2021). Leave no trace, willful unknowing, and implications from the ethics of sustainability for solution-focused practice outdoors. *Journal of Solution Focused Practices*, 5(2), 7.

Norcross, J. C., & Lambert, M. J. (2011). Psychotherapy relationships that work II. *Psychotherapy*, 48(1), 4–8. https://doi.org/10.1037/a0022180

Rogers, C. R. (1957). The necessary and sufficient conditions of therapeutic personality change. *Journal of Consulting Psychology*, 21(2), 95–103. https://doi.org/10.1037/h0045357

Rosen, K. (2020). *Troubled: The failed promise of America's behavioral programs*. Little A.

Rosenzweig, S. (1936). Some implicit common factors in diverse methods of psychotherapy. American Journal of Orthopsychiatry, 6(3), 412–415. https://doi.org/10.1111/j.1939-0025.1936.tb05248.x

Russell, K. C., & Farnum, J. (2004). A concurrent model of the wilderness therapy process. *Journal of Adventure Education & Outdoor Learning*, 4(1), 39–55. https://doi.org/10.1080/14729670485200411

Shennan, G. (2019). *Solution-focused practice: Effective communication to facilitate change* (2nd ed.) Red Globe Press.

Smith, M. L., & Glass, G. V. (1977). Meta-analysis of psychotherapy outcome studies. American Psychologist, 32(9), 752–760. https://doi.org/10.1037/0003-066X.32.9.752

Stigsdotter, U. K., Corazon, S. S., Sidenius, U., Nyed, P. K., Larsen, H. B., & Fjorback, L. O. (2018). Efficacy of nature-based therapy for individuals with stress-related illnesses: Randomised controlled trial. *The British Journal of Psychiatry*, 213(1), 404–411. https://doi.org/10.1192/bjp.2018.2

Strupp, H. H., & Hadley, S. W. (1979). Specific vs nonspecific factors in psychotherapy: A controlled study of outcome. *Archives of General Psychiatry*, 36(10), 1125–1136. https://doi.org/10.1001/archpsyc.1979.01780100095009

Tucker, A. R., Javorski, S., Tracy, J., & Beale, B. (2013). The use of adventure therapy in community-based mental health: Decreases in problem severity among youth clients. *Child & Youth Care Forum*, 42(2), 155–179. https://doi.org/10.1007/s10566-012-9190-x

Wampold, B. E. (2007). Psychotherapy: The humanistic (and effective) treatment. American Psychologist, 62(8), 857–873. https://doi.org/10.1037/0003-066X.62.8.857

Wampold, B. E., & Brown, G. S. J. (2005). Estimating variability in outcomes attributable to therapists: A naturalistic study of outcomes in managed care. *Journal of Consulting and Clinical Psychology*, 73(5), 914–923. https://doi.org/10.1037/0022-006X.73.5.914

Wampold, B. E., & Imel, Z. E. (2015). *The great psychotherapy debate: The evidence for what makes psychotherapy work* (2nd ed.) Routledge.

3

Tools for the Solution-Focused Practitioner

"People are just as wonderful as sunsets if you let them be. When I look at a sunset, I don't find myself saying, 'Soften the orange a bit on the right hand corner.' I don't try to control a sunset. I watch with awe as it unfolds."

Carl Rogers (1980, p. 22)

If you have read about or have adopted a solution-focused approach, much of this book will have a familiar ring. There are, however, aspects in this chapter which build on what we refer to as classic solution-focused brief therapy. Critiques of solution-focused practice include that it is simply a series of specific techniques with goals pursued at the expense of the therapeutic alliance to be delivered at distinct moments of a therapeutic interaction (Wettersten et al., 2005). Essentially, a computer could do it. Goddard (1996) argued changes made through solution-focused practice were superficial. The practitioner's intuition is not used enough, the engagement is insufficiently authentic, and the lack of psychological insight places action over reflection. Some have found the language overly intellectual and to discount economic, societal, and cultural oppression. Ratner et al. (2012) reviewed these and other criticisms and deftly batted them away. The heart and art of solution-focused therapy is in the assumptions practitioners make about those they work with and what works in their therapeutic interactions.

In this chapter, we describe the positionality and stance adopted in this approach, followed by the tools used by solution-focused practitioners. While there are specific questions we ask and certain methods, like adopting a future focus, so much of the cash value is in how we see and perceive those we work with. This also changes how we view their participation during one of our outdoor sessions. For example, is a young person court mandated to an outdoor expedition not an active, self-determining participant? Of course they are. We want to know about their preferred future and provide an

DOI: 10.4324/9781003217558-4

opportunity for that person to witness themselves at their best. Like all models of therapy, the way we perceive the therapeutic interaction is grounded in various philosophical positions and cultural contexts. Ultimately, co-adventurers should leave us better able to cope in their lives, with more agency, self-efficacy, and hope than when they joined us.

I (Will) studied social work in the United States before continuing my studies in Australia. While I used the term therapy and even psychotherapy in the United States, Australian social workers may refer to their work as counseling, or resist both terms altogether. Cultural context is inexplicably tied to our approach and has to be given due attention and respect, even if just to reduce confusion over what exactly we are talking about.

Working throughout Europe, I (Stephan) was educated on the use of the word "therapy" and how it can be taken to mean many more things than expected. Something is lost in translation. In Latvia, little seemed to make sense about adventure therapy until the word "counseling" was substituted for therapy and the penny dropped. Similarly, the word *healing* in the context of talking therapy can be problematic. Language and what words are assumed to mean is fundamental to understanding. The philosopher Wittgenstein's work was influential to the early solution-focused workers (McKergow, 2021) and his view that language is a fluid interactional practice to get things done has been a lesson learned many times. It is always wise to check the meaning of words and not to assume understanding is mutually agreed. There are, however, some words solution-focused practitioners avoid (see Appendix C). We adopted a version of spelling for this text familiar to readers with American English rather than British English, though it is possible some colloquialisms from the European, Australian, and US use of English have made an appearance. We can only hope our meaning is understood in print.

Kazdin (2000) argued in the *Encyclopaedia of Psychology* that all models of counseling and psychotherapy are informed by specific philosophical positions. For instance, each type of therapy comes with its own theoretical perceptions and techniques for working with people based on that worldview. Examining how theory informs therapeutic modalities helps to understand the emergence of solution-focused approaches and our considerations for taking this practice outdoors.

Though Sigmund Freud bears the brunt of many therapy jokes, cultural context played a major role in the development of his psychoanalysis (Frank & Frank, 1991). Freud lived in a male-dominated society that placed high value on individual success and achievement. People feared too much openness could expose a man's weakness. It was also believed that if someone maintained too much concern for the welfare of other people, they would be unable to achieve their individual goals. Behavior was assumed to be conjured from fantasy, such as incest, and was seldom discussed. Freud often invited his patients to speak freely, using the technique of free associations, where a client would talk about anything and everything that entered their mind, even if these topics were potentially humiliating. In this case, it is no wonder Freud often sat behind the patient, who was lying on the couch facing the ceiling.

Things changed when these theories and modalities crossed the Atlantic and embedded themselves in American psychology, which was less of an authoritarian system. Where Freud's clients were instructed to lay on a couch making no direct eye contact with their therapist, America's therapy recipients began to sit directly across from their clinician, maintaining eye contact where appropriate. The therapist became more friendly and supportive, as opposed to a distant, all knowing, authoritative father figure.

It is important to consider various models of counseling and psychotherapy and views of outdoor therapies as a *cultural enterprise*, as recommended by Frank and Frank (1991). As we discuss in this chapter, cultural context helps to construct the theories we lean on for justification of our solution-focused outdoor work. First, we consider how culture impacts perceptions of outdoor settings.

Naturalists John Muir and Henry David Thoreau spent most of their lives playing in the American outdoors. They are well regarded for quotes and passages about *preserving the wilderness*. The word wilderness stems from the Old English *wild dēor*, or wild deer. A Google search will tell you that a wilderness is defined as "an uncultivated, uninhabited, and inhospitable region" (n.p.). This construction of the wild discounts the Traditional Custodians of these lands, whether they are the Lakota Sioux, Inuit, Cherokee, or any other group of Indigenous peoples. One of us has been to Antarctica, maybe the only "true" wilderness given this definition, except perhaps for deep caves where the other author spends much of his time. Reflecting on terminology and the nature-human kinship (Harper & Dobud, 2020), we find it critical for outdoor practitioners to reflect on their relationship with the outdoors.

The Australian Association for Bush Adventure Therapy, Inc. (AABAT, 2021) acknowledged that many practitioners in Australia may describe their work as *wilderness therapy*, as we too have in the past. However, the history of bush adventure therapy requires unpacking to understand how cultural context informs the way we perceive our work. According to AABAT's website, the new "terminology recognises that 'wilderness' may be seen as a colonizing term (implying 'people-free') that ignores the Indigenous presence in the land. The new title of Bush Adventure Therapy emphasizes relationships with the natural environment in our work and practice" (para. 2).

During a presentation at the 7th International Adventure Therapy Conference in Denver, Colorado, the late Leiv Einer Gabriellsen and his Norwegian counterpart Carina Ribe Fernee described their grassroots efforts in establishing a new wilderness therapy program at their local Sørlandet Hospital. Raising their hand, a guest in the audience asked Leiv about public liability and other logistical issues, such as running expeditions on public land. Leiv described how in Norway there are little to no laws about land use for camping. You can camp freely on someone's farm as long as you are a certain distance from their residence. All government-led search and rescue efforts, even if requiring additional resources or helicopters, are free; even for the tourist lost in a blizzard. We learned from our Norwegian colleagues about the value of encouraging people to explore the beautiful outdoor environments Norway has to offer. Cultural context influences outdoor therapy endeavors. In Norway, it was not surprising to see most of the adolescents arrive to their expedition with their own gear. While working in Alaska, many of the participants knew more about the local forests and animals than the guides from the lower 48 US states. We encourage practitioners to reflect on their relationship to the outdoors and the specific models of therapy they deliver, appreciating the cultural enterprise that is therapy and the assumptions they make about the outdoors.

As our worldview informs the narrative we tell about natural settings and outdoor environments, so too does it inform our view of psychotherapy and how it works. Thus far, we have briefly examined how culture finds its way into the construction of therapy services. Next, we examine how the philosophy of social construction, as well as other philosophical orientations, informs what we know about solution-focused practices.

Getting Philosophical

One strength to solution-focused practice is how we address the theoretical orientation that informs this work. As we have examined thus far, there are inherent limitations to the medical model within the helping professions, yet it retains a strong hold on the field. The medical model in therapy, in its most simplistic form, is the belief that with the right diagnosis, a practitioner can choose an empirically supported therapy to treat that disorder, like taking antibiotics for an infection. While this is overly simple, this informs the most influential research being done in our field (Clark et al., 2004; Wampold & Imel, 2015). The social context, and cultural influence as we described, is all but missing in this irreconcilable view of therapy as medicine. A solution-focused approach is grounded in a different view of helping. We are informed by social construction, a workable theory for how people make meaning.

In the late 1800s, philosophers around the world argued that social scientists should borrow research methodologies from the physical sciences, like chemistry, physics, and biology (Smith, 1983). This was referred to as *positivism*, a philosophical stance that reality is only recognizable if it can be objectively and scientifically proven, requiring some form of mathematical proof. As you can imagine, this created heated debates about religious or spiritual experiences. If it cannot be mathematically tested, is it real? I (Stephan) sense there is a debate to be had around a pragmatic use of imaginary numbers, though we can leave that for now.

While many would argue otherwise, this positivist orientation has informed much of our view of mental health. We have a growing book, the *Diagnostic and Statistical Manual of Mental Disorders* (APA, 2013), now in its fifth edition, and government- or insurance-approved lists of treatments for addressing these diagnoses (SAMHSA, 2021). In order for your therapy of choice to join such databases, you will need multiple randomized clinical trials, using quantitative clinical measures to prove your therapy is efficacious, cost-effective, and safe. Researchers at the Outdoor Behavioral Healthcare Center (2021) have been hard at work to achieve this stamp of approval for wilderness therapy in the United States.

Here lies the problem. More treatments, rigorous training, or clinical supervision have not led to a single percentage improvement of therapy outcomes (Miller et al., 2013). This is not due to a lack of effort. It is because the philosophical stance informing what we know about mental health and the treatment of psychological distress stems from the "hard" sciences. Consider this thought experiment. You are sitting with a client at the top of a mountain. You are both exhausted, drinking water while munching on trail mix. Your client begins telling you about a religious experience they had as a child. You, of no religious orientation, begin questioning what happened to lead to this experience. Was your client brainwashed at a young age? Maybe she was hallucinating? Is it related to trauma, or some other neuromyth, neurobabble, or pseudoscience (Misheva, 2020)? After all, there is little scientific or mathematical evidence to support the "truth" surrounding the religion she believes in.

This was a concern from opposing philosophers in the late 1800s. The push towards a mathematical view of human life loses the entire complexity of lived experience (Dobud & Cavanaugh, 2020). Said another way, if we have such little understanding of mundane human experience, how are we ever going to understand rich phenomena, such as sitting with someone describing a religious experience on top of a mountain or working therapeutically with someone from a drastically different culture with values directly opposed to ours? This is why a solution-focus, though artfully basic in technique, requires strong theoretical grounding. This discipline is more important than the techniques themselves, as this stance can work without asking for exceptions to the problem, or using the miracle question with the perfect verbiage and tone of voice, or even saying much at all (Natynczuk, 2021). We begin with a brief examination of *social construction*, as the foundational theory for solution-focused practice and how we approach this work outdoors. Though first we would like to say something about some finer considerations underlying our approach.

Co-Adventuring for Co-Construction

Social constructionists discard any notion of objective truth that is merely waiting to be discovered. In constructionism, "knowledge is established through the meanings attached to the phenomena studied" (Krauss, 2005, p. 759). The main tenant of this philosophy is that reality is constructed, never discovered. Thus, it is different for everyone and the methods of inquiry dictate what there is to be found. For example, data from qualitative interviews with practitioners suggest it is the healing power of nature contributing to client change in outdoor therapy (Naor & Mayseless, 2021). When we use quantitative measures to assess how nature contributes to outcome, we find little evidence to support such claims (Dobud & Harper, 2018). It is not whether one method is better than the next. The question is how the method itself directs the inquirer to certain conclusions.

It is in the outdoor therapy interaction that meaning is given to experience. The outdoor solution-focused adventure is itself a new opportunity for co-adventurers to construct meaning about their preferred future, ideally one in which the problem that brought the person to therapy is no longer present. Through asking detailed and thoughtful questions, participants provide specific descriptions and attach specific meaning to any outdoor experience.

Peeters and Ringer (2020) described how outdoor therapy practitioners should take care in naming the experiential activities they facilitate. Using the example of a "trust fall," in which a person may be blindfolded while falling backwards only to be caught by their peers, they argued that this name takes away from the participants' ability to freely construct meaning. In fact, just telling them, "We're going to do a trust fall," prescribes the meaning you intend that they construct. Instead, the solution-focused practitioner maintains an openness to experience, knowing that with careful questioning, co-adventurers construct any meaning they wish. Adopting the stance of not knowing, practitioners inquire with their outdoor therapy participants about the meaning they are making. We trust participants to produce or construct their own personal meaning. This alone makes outdoor therapy so rich and we expand on this below.

In our clinical work, we have noticed that when we establish an as equitable therapeutic relationship as possible, our co-adventurers will let us know what experiences or conversations have been particularly meaningful. For instance, while working with a group of adults diagnosed with severe and persistent mental illnesses, some described hikes near the river as a time for normalcy. Others shared that they felt peace in the outdoor setting, while some enjoyed the exercise. Some mostly enjoyed the talking. We agree with Krauss' (2005) definition that meaning is "the cognitive categories that make up one's view of reality and with which actions are defined" (p. 762). New experiences generate and enrich meaning, while meaning also provides clarification and guidance for an experience. Put simply, *new doing makes for new thinking*. The reason we *must* partner with our co-adventurers is because it is entirely possible that any therapy service we provide can leave a person demoralized, invalidated, or worse off. If we treat every therapy recipient as capable of constructing their own meaning from experience, we can avoid being overly prescriptive, truly trusting they are experts in their own life. This can be a leap of faith for some practitioners in negotiating and applying just the right amount of control for safety reasons in outdoor work.

As solution-focused practitioners, we refrain from general descriptions of cause and effect, or generic hypotheses, and instead attempt to account for the "often taken-for-granted" experiences within therapy outdoors (Polkinghorne, 1992). Theories of constructionism emphasize that knowledge is generated through experience, without the necessity of mathematical predictions or law-like bodies of knowledge.

Where solution-focused practice is mischaracterized necessitates further examination. As we have stated, the solution-focused stance is not about prescribing solutions, nor a specific set of techniques delivered void of context, perhaps following some sort of flow chart of tools. We certainly avoid the prescription of exercises and games designed to treat and cure a diagnosis. Where some, such as Bannink (2010), have argued for a solution-focused cognitive behavioral therapy, we want to stress that the approach we are describing in this book requires a strong, disciplined, and regimented philosophy. Some practitioners have viewed solution-focused approaches as a buffet of techniques or questions, perhaps to incorporate some solution-focused tools into their regularly preferred modality. Sure, there are many techniques worthy of implementation. That said, we urge you to reflect on the philosophical stance you bring to your work. If there is not one, you may risk unwillfully imposing your values and worldviews on those who seek your service (Natynczuk & Dobud, 2021).

The seductive allure of solution-focused techniques is in the deceptive ease of their administration. We have heard, "I *do* ask the miracle question, and then I get on with my dialectical behavioral therapy (DBT) work." First, of course we are thrilled you are eliciting the preferred future of who you are working with. Second, the concern is how you work with it. We have no opposition to DBT. It works, and works well. However, reflection is required to rationalize how two opposing philosophical stances can be used interchangeably. DBT can be quite a directive therapy, where solution-focused is more client-directed. Additionally, there are concerns about the psychological and emotional depth at which the solution-focused practitioner works. Borrowed tools are often underused. We have witnessed practitioners using the tomorrow question, only to quickly move on to the next question without significantly exploring the details of the response. Solution-focused practitioners are encouraged to respectfully probe to expand the narrative around what the client will notice. The more detail the better, as we will uncover finer details of change that are implementable.

For example, we avoid "reading between the lines" of our co-adventurers' lived experience. Ratner et al. (2012) have found this stance has led to arguments about whether maintaining a solution-focus leaves therapeutic encounters firmly positioned on the surface, ignoring the emotional or psychological depth required for effective psychotherapy. Consider how many of us are taught to interpret the emotions of those we work with, such as when someone is crying during a group therapy session. Miller and de Shazer (2000) wrote, in response to such critique, that therapists have needlessly constructed a field that "treats emotions as abstract entities about which some therapists are uniquely knowledgeable" (p. 70). Inner experiences, such as a participant describing feeling like a burden during a session in a canoe, should not be explored in isolation to social context and action. Consider the example of someone crying. One can cry tears of joy or sadness, or when chopping an onion. We work with people based solely on the information and responses they provide, and avoid dichotomies, such as surface versus depth. Emotions are not separated from social context and action, and despite our training, we do not approach people as experts in their lived experience. How could we possibly know what others experience? A lucky guess is the best we could hope for, so to be sure remain humble and respectful. Evidence is everything.

Instead, we remain vigilant and grounded in our philosophical positions. As recommended by Selekman (2005), we refer to our position based on a series of *theoretical assumptions*. We unpack these assumptions below. Practitioners from all theoretical backgrounds maintain perceptions about the people they work with. As solution-focused practitioners, we are conscious, careful, and intentional about the assumptions we bring to practice. These assumptions are grounded in theories of social construction, pragmatism, humanism, and self-determination. Just as Rogers (1980) described his example of viewing clients as unfolding sunsets we have no motivation to change or alter, we use the assumptions below to remain diligent and disciplined in this humanistic stance.

Theoretical Assumptions

Being solution-focused is non-normalizing. Everyone is regarded as their own expert on what they want from life and participants are viewed as capable of constructing meaning throughout our outdoor experiences. If they are not experiencing any benefit from our work together, we view this as an area that is actionable on behalf of the practitioner, not as due to any fault of the participant. How we perceive people as active participants is central. While they may experience psychological distress, or be in trouble due to their own problematic behavior, we begin by establishing a partnership for change, based on their best hopes for our work together and for their own preferred future. What meaning will be constructed throughout our adventures, interactions, and experiences? We have to wait and see. A true *adventure* is an undertaking with an uncertain outcome.

The following sections explore client motivation, resistance, how we can co-create a culture of competence, their perception of their best self, solution-forced orientations, and, similar to motivational interviewing, how we listen for change talk.

Do Unmotivated Clients Exist?

When I (Will) started my practice in Adelaide, South Australia, I was thrilled, and honestly quite shocked, when the first mother called me to book a session for her son. His father had recently died and her son was completely disengaged from school and was now self-harming. He had seen psychologists and psychiatrists, but the mother really just wanted him to see someone different. My office was under renovation so I agreed to meet at a local park. I arrived 15 minutes early so I could relax and prepare for the session. I was very nervous that this was the *first* co-adventurer of my new business endeavor. He did not get out of the car. The mother got out and spoke with me. I did not want him to think we were gossiping about him. I looked in the window and knew the band on his sweatshirt. "Wow! Is that Refused?" I asked. "I can't believe you know them! Are you into that type of music?" This is how our conversation went for the next few minutes through the car window. He got out of the car and we sat under a large gum tree and talked about music. I snuck in questions about his best hopes and got an idea of his preferred future. Next session, he brought music for us to listen to. His best hopes for the session were to connect with an adult who was not a teacher or his parent. The following week, his mother rang and said he had gone to school for the first time in over a year.

Years later, while sitting in the canoe with that same young person (now in university) I asked about what happened. "Hey, I never really asked you this. When you finally went to school, what happened?" He responded that no one ever asked what he wanted. He said every worker just spoke about school (the problem) or his father's death (another problem). The research is clear that finding consensus between a practitioner and client about the purpose of their work together is vital (Norcross & Lambert, 2011). Practitioners can struggle when prescribing a purpose without understanding a person's best hopes. At best, this is guesswork. At worst, arrogance. It is important to consider each client's motivation. Assuming they are unmotivated provides a safe and easy escape for us out of the therapeutic relationship. It is entirely possible that we, as helping professionals, have contributed to our clients' lack of faith that therapy, of any kind, will resolve the problems that brought them to us in the first place. While some clients are referred to as involuntary or mandated, we remain vigilant in exploring their motivation. If anything, this may stress that we take their lived experience seriously.

Nearly every solution-focused session begins with some sort of contracting to establish what we are working on that day. "At the end of our time together, what would you notice that told you it was useful?" is a question that goes straight to the essence of what a client wants from the interaction. Sometimes people are sent to therapy by third parties. The client turns up perhaps because they want their parents, teacher, social worker, or youth justice worker to leave them alone for a while. Solution-focused practitioners may ask, "Given that you have arrived here, how can this time we have together be useful for you?"

Hill (2007) found that many practitioners felt adolescents were the most difficult to approach therapeutically. While we agree that we have seen adolescent after adolescent walk through our doors certain our work will align with their parents, school, previous therapists, or the court systems, we have found that if we want to leave our clients feeling invalidated, we should not ask about their motivation. Instead, we follow along the work of Sparks et al. (2007) who stressed the importance of positioning the adolescent as central to the change process. We also perceive the client as central to defining any therapeutic aims and progress. Others have termed this co-production (Nature, 2021).

There Is No Such Thing as an Unmotivated Client

If a client decides not to engage in an activity or therapeutic task, we avoid over-theorizing about why. Their lack of engagement is not due to their trauma or resistance to therapy, it is most often due to an issue in our therapeutic relationship or a lack of consensus about the purpose of the interaction. This can get tricky when we are working with people pressured to see us by another person, but the art remains establishing an idea for the client's preferred future, providing experiences of success and mastery in the outdoors, and exploring how the meaning made from the outdoor therapy experience can impact a person's life when they head home.

Resistance Is Not a Useful Concept

Steve de Shazer's first draft of his paper, "Death to resistance," was first submitted to a journal in 1979. It was rejected. It took 17 rejections and six revisions before finding its publication in 1984. de Shazer (1989) followed up on his original paper insisting "the concept of resistance was a bad idea for therapists to have in their heads" (p. 227). He argued that what once began as a metaphor describing that it is "as if" a client is resisting morphed into a certainty that a client "is" being resistant. He goes on to describe the problem:

> Resistance is a peculiar concept. In essence, it meant that the thera-
> pist and client/patient had a fight and then, when the therapist won
> and resistance was overcome, the loser of the fight got to go home
> changed – which is really what the client came to therapy for in the
> first place. So losing was winning.
>
> (p. 228)

We have worked with what many classically define as *involuntary* clients. We acknowledge young people can be "resistant" to the idea of coming to therapy, no matter the type or whether indoors or out. There is often a problematic behavior central to the referral, such as drug use, self-harming, problematic eating, or criminal activity. When we label those we work with as resistant, we enter into the win-lose debate de Shazer (1989) was illuminating all those years ago.

Consider which of these statements you have heard in your outdoor therapy work, or which you might hear in the future. "Steve… he is just not engaged in the program." "I know he is a nice guy, but Bill has just not accepted why he is here." "Sally has not hit rock bottom, and until she does, she will not benefit from the work." "How can he change if he can't acknowledge his sins?" These statements place the sole responsibility of engagement on the client and exclude ourselves from the therapeutic relationship.

More bad therapy seldom leads to good therapy. Practitioners are encouraged to partner with those disengaged to find something different they can do together, as opposed to doing more of the same. Dobud's (2020) qualitative research found many participants in US wilderness therapy programs were punished due to a lack of engagement. Some were thrown from their sleeping bags into the snow, and others required to start the program over again. Resistance is not a useful concept because of the win-lose scenario de Shazer (1989) described.

Creating a Culture of Competence

The solution-focused approach draws on strengths and competences to show that a client has their own personal tools for change at hand. It seems all too easy to forget one's strengths and the many things we are competent at, as if celebrating being good at something is almost socially unacceptable. We might start a session by asking what a client is good at, what they like doing in their free time, or what they enjoy doing the most when they get a chance? If we had examples of these helpful attributes at hand, what difference would more make? Exploring the difference strengths and exceptions make with a scale can help generate hope for change, especially in conjunction with remembering instances when those strengths helped make a useful difference. Another way to consider such instances is to explore exceptions: times when whatever has brought the client to therapy did not exist. To ask a client to remember themselves as competent and capable helps break a pattern of behavior that might contribute to being stuck in a problem.

Practitioners communicate how important co-adventurers are to the group and provide opportunities for choice regularly. If a practitioner rolls an ankle, or worse, the participants may be required to pitch in and help. Aim for co-adventurers to experience the *Crucial C's* (adapted from Lew & Bettern, 1996):

- Feeling a sense of **connection** with their practitioner and/or other participants.
- Having the **capability** to participate fully in the outdoor therapy session, even when adapted to specific needs.
- Feeling valued by those they interact with and that what they do **counts** and will make a difference in the group.
- Having **courage**.

The climate of competence provides an experience where participants can experience exceptions to life's problems during the therapy encounter. After carefully facilitating the experience outdoors, solution-focused practitioners ask carefully crafted questions to examine what meaning people have (re) discovered from the experiencing of their competent self. A resource in the field manual provides a framework for practitioners to conceptualize outdoor therapy experiences using the Crucial C's (see Appendix D).

Provide Clients a Chance to See and Be Their Best Selves

Talking about ourselves at our best often feels uncomfortable for first-time solution-focused clients, though it is a useful way to build confidence. Occasionally, clients find it difficult to talk of themselves as someone who achieves. Perhaps they do not have the vocabulary or imagination to describe what someone else would notice when they were at their best. It is, however, safe to assume they have an experience worth sharing when they have been at their best. An alternative way for the practitioner to gather such evidence is to provide an opportunity for a client to be at their best for hours at a time, a whole day, or even a number of days in succession through an outdoor activity, journey, or multi-day expedition.

Jeanne attended a wilderness therapy expedition for young people impacted by cancer. Like the other adolescents in her group, she only recently finished her third bout of chemotherapy when she saw the invitation to the adventure tacked to the corkboard in the hospital's hallway. She was nervous. She felt physically weak and questioned whether she was up for the seven-day white water rafting program. However, she shared during the program all the aspects of her formative teenage years cancer had taken from her. There was no prom, no first kiss, and her love of gymnastics was put on hold. During the program, however, she was allowed to be wild. She remembers being given something she never knew was missing. Through the adventure, she saw herself at her best, able to build strong relationships with others who shared similar lived experiences, and was given respite to her identity as a cancer patient.

Solution-Forced

When practitioners prescribe goals or believe they know what is best for their clients, they risk becoming *solution-forced* (Nylund & Corsiglia, 1994; Thomas, 2007). Being deceptively simple, practitioners can misread solution-focused brief therapy. We must keep our assumptions about how we view clients, change, and problems in our conscious awareness. Clients already have the resources to change and we work towards their preferred future. Exceptions to problems always exist and more exceptions are lived experientially during outdoor therapy sessions. Solution-*forced* practitioners fail to adhere to this orientation, and instead are waiting patiently at the finish line while their client is left at the starting gate feeling invalidated.

Nylund and Corsiglia (1994) argued that to become solution-*forced*, practitioners need to practice one or more of the following:

1. Permit the client to only engage in "solution talk." Indicate to the client that the problem should not be discussed at all.
2. Attend to exceptions that do not make a difference to the client.
3. Fail to co-construct a goal; do not seek the client's goals for therapy. (p. 6)

We avoid allowing our theories of change or pathology to interfere with attending to a person's individual needs and preferences. We risk becoming solution-forced when we believe our work is more special than anyone else's simply due to the setting it takes place in or the interventions we deliver. The case example below demonstrates how practitioners can easily fall into the solution-*forced* trap.

During her residential wilderness therapy stay, Mary-Anne's therapist noticed that she was smiling more than any day before. When asked about what was happening, Mary-Anne said she felt a bit better and slightly more connected to the group. Enthusiastically, the practitioner congratulated Mary-Anne and began a line of questioning asking how she was able to be happy. "You don't get it. I'm not happy. This place fucking sucks. It is just a little bit better than yesterday." When talking to one of her peers in the group, another practitioner overheard Mary-Anne voicing the agitation of being forced into change because her therapist saw one little smile. The purpose of the expedition was missing, any therapeutic alliance was absent, and the small exception of a smile did not make any difference to Mary-Anne.

Solution-focused practice is mischaracterized by the notion that we *never* talk about problems. We have to legitimize a person's concerns and collaborate with their truth. Nylund and Corsiglia (1994) presented what they called the Five D's for avoiding solution-focused work, building on the earlier list of how to be solution-*forced*:

- Do not acknowledge or validate the client's experience of the problem.
- Do ask questions in a mechanical or instrumental manner without tailoring and attuning to the emotional context, pacing of the discussion or client's body language.
- Do search for and argue for exceptions that make no difference to the client.
- Do view yourself as the expert therapist and pursue what you think is best, not the client's goals or preferred future.
- Do not construct a therapeutic climate of respect, curiosity, transparency, and openness.

Becoming solution-forced is a trap any practitioner can fall into. Practitioners will notice in the field manual (see Appendix E) many documents which can be used in the field or supervision to help with keeping their eyes on the important assumptions that facilitate collaborative working relationships.

Hope

Experiencing the absence of hope is perhaps the lowest a person can get. Working therapeutically with people presenting themselves with an absence of hope is probably some of the toughest, most challenging and serious work a practitioner will ever do. Hope can be defined as "to want something to happen or to be true, and usually have a good reason to think that it might." This definition from the online Cambridge English Dictionary will look very familiar to solution-focused practitioners; it is what we work towards with every client. Indeed, every session begins with "What are your best hopes for our work together?" – an invitation to think big into the future. Generating hope is not the special reserve of solution-focused practice; all good therapy should generate hope (Kelley et al., 2010). However, hope is at the center of solution-focused practice. Among the many examples in the literature, Shennan's (2019) chapter on *Acknowledgement and Possibility* is a good read for those interested in some of the finer details of hope in solution-focused practices.

Tools for the Solution-Focused Practitioner

We would like to visit some of the tools in the solution-focused practitioner's backpack as we shall refer to them from time to time and address their application to outdoor therapy sessions. We aim to gently guide co-adventurers to a point in the future when they no longer need to attend our sessions; essentially plotting a history for that future. Whatever tool we use, it is important to ask "What else?" The first few responses are the easy ones. As more detail is requested, clients have to work harder. The more specific the detail, the easier it becomes to find small, realizable, things to change in order to make a difference: the client has to do this for themselves. They arrive at the solution with only the most gentle and curious guidance from our questioning.

We hope you forgive us a certain amount of repetition as we talk about these tools. We have repeated ourselves so each tool can be viewed on its own, without having to read the whole chapter each time. We omitted transcripts of sessions, firstly because we did not want to write a customary solution-focused book, secondly to keep the chapter from getting too long, and thirdly because there are plenty of transcripts of solution-focused conversations in the literature, for example George et al. (1990), McKergow (2021), Ratner et al. (2012), Shennan (2019), and Yusuf (2021).

First and Third Person Perspectives

First person perspectives are the responses we receive from our questions to the client. They offer insight into the hopes, expectations, aspirations, strengths, motivations, and opportunities directly from the client. We might also inquire what others would notice when something is going better for the person we are working with. These are third person perspectives. We might ask what a significant person who cares for the client's wellbeing would notice if our work together was heading in the right direction. Additionally, we can ask them to look out for signs of hope. Asking "What else?" elicits the finer details, perhaps five, ten, or more times until we find instances and exceptions to work with.

For example, while processing a team-building exercise with a group of young adults in a residential facility focused on substance use, a participant shares that she thought effective communication and listening skills were important to successfully completing the group task. The solution-focused practitioner may ask what difference the listening made, focusing attention onto what made the group successful. Then, the practitioner orients the questions towards the clients' preferred future. "If listening is important here, what difference would it make when you leave this facility? What about next week? Tomorrow? In one hour?"

We can also ask what a third party might notice. "If you were listening more attentively, what would your partner notice?" Follow up with "What difference would it make?" Practitioners ask for signs of change rather than a list of actions. Actions and tasks can lead to creating a list of things that never get done. Especially so if our client sees them as unimportant. Actions and tasks can evoke a list of the same old actions that our client might think are expected, ought to be done, or in others' best interests. We should be alert to lists of actions as the top of the slippery slope to solution-forced or even coercive practice.

Scaling Questions

Scales usually run from 0 to 10 and focus on a person's confidence or competence to bring about change. Ideally, clients will help define the description of the limits. Traditionally, 0 is the worse something could be, or its absence, and 10 the best. Somewhere in between 0 and 10 is where people score their current position. There is also a point that is good enough. Concentrating on the score provided, clients are invited to describe as many observations of what makes up that score, or what contributes to that number, as they can.

Sally, a 78-year-old widow who recently moved into an aged care facility, engages weekly with a solution-focused horticultural therapist. While planting new vegetables in the front garden, the therapist asks Sally to rate on a scale of 0 to 10 how confident she has felt about the transition to the facility improving. Sally reported being a 3. She said she missed her partner and felt lonely in the supportive living environment. The practitioner asked for evidence as to why she is at a 3. "Well, I am able to garden, which I liked to do at home, and I know I'm a pretty strong person," she responded. The practitioner took note of these exceptions and inquired what Sally would notice if things progressed up the scale to a 4, or even higher, asking "What else?" to detail the small signs of change.

We are helping our client to record anything that helps them to be at their best, evidencing their strengths and resources. We inquire what they would notice more of as they moved up the scale; even just a little bit, maybe a full point, maybe half a point if more appropriate. Ask which is preferred and gently press for as much detail as possible. Scoring on a scale gives us a measured unit to later compare change from session to session and is thus evidence of change clients achieved for themselves.

However, here are some notes of caution. Scaling questions are helpful for collecting people's evidence of exceptions to their troubles and illustrating they are moving in the direction of their preferred future. It is often the case that scales are used superficially, though their value is found in their use to uncover the smallest observations of things that are noticed to be changeable (Bliss & Bray, 2009). This requires a gentle, respectful persistence with a genuine curiosity for detail. It is not always necessary for the practitioner to actually know the number the client thinks of. They can keep that to themselves. The practitioner asks what the client notices that contributes to that number, collecting as much detail as can be given, then asks something like, "When you move up the scale, even just a small nudge up the scale, what will you see more of that begins to make a difference?"

We imagine advocates for experiential processing to be constructing ideas for encouraging more active bodily engagement when using scaling questions. You might use a slackline, climbing wall, or pebbles along a stream to craft innovative scales. You might use scaling questions after an activity and encourage the participants to repeat the activity supposing they are one point higher on the scale. Scales are often critiqued as banal tools for the lowly psychotherapy: "On a scale from 1 to 10, how are you feeling today?"

Scales, and the many tools we provide throughout the book, require careful artistry and are only as powerful as how they are delivered, received, and processed.

Difference

Asking, with respectful curiosity, "What difference would that make?" can be directed at our client to explore how changes in their behavior can be received by those in the person's life. Difference in anything is a change worth noting. During an outdoor therapy experience, a co-adventurer may experience an exception to what brought them to therapy. For example, while rock climbing, a client says, "I have never been well organized but today I was able to take care of all of the gear and learn how it works." While this statement may appear surface level, we assure you it is not. We may ask, "If you were organized like this at home, what difference would that make?" Ask what others would notice, and so on. The more detail the better.

Inquiring about differences creates a bridge between the outdoor therapy setting and lived experience. These questions help co-adventurers to link their moments of success and mastery, their experience of the climate of competence, and any exceptions to their life at elsewhere. Transfer of learning is difficult when therapy is conducted away from a person's community (Harper et al., 2019). These questions are used to improve sustainability and consolidate gains made during a session.

The Great Instead

Most people come to us with very real problems. Substance use, depression, anxiety, trauma, abuse, neglect, and family conflict are the usual suspects. There are times when asking about someone's best hopes that they stress they simply want one of these problems to go away. "I don't want to be depressed anymore," a 45-year-old veteran may pronounce. If we accept this preferred future and contract to work on no longer being depressed, we risk adopting a problem focus (Ratner et al., 2012). We will focus on the person's depression, eliciting information about what it looks like, the length of its presence, and its etymology.

When provided with statements such as these, we may ask, "Instead of feeling depressed, what might you notice instead?" Or if they have flashbacks to bad times, "Tell me about flashbacks to the good things you've done."

This type of question directs conversation away from problem talk. Talking about problems keeps problems alive and can lead to being stuck. Some may be tempted to problem solve on behalf of the client. When a participant wants to talk about their problems, it is important we listen. We do not want them left feeling invalidated. We do, however, gently guide discussion towards their preferred future by noticing exceptions and instances of their preferred future being possible. Only when the time is right.

As the participant describes experiences that exist *instead* of depression, we ask how our time together can make a difference. We inquire about what they will notice during and after the session when they live out this difference. If we are inviting this veteran on a caving program, we may ask, "What will you notice that brings you joy (instead of depression)?" or "What would you be pleased to notice during our time in the cave?" These questions invite real-time possibilities and collaboration. They energize the co-adventurer by increasing hope for a future with something other than depression.

Powerful Suppose

Suppose is possibly the most powerful word in the solution-focused toolkit. In many ways, the future is an imaginary place. We can only make predictions, so imagining a better future is an option we have for talking about a time when whatever brought our client to therapy no longer exists. Additionally, we can frame questions after certain experiences using the word suppose. For example, after a session walking along the beach with a client, a practitioner asks, "You mentioned feeling at peace when you're listening to the water. Suppose you felt this same peace at home, what difference would that make?" Wait for the answer, then follow up with something like "What would you (and/or others) notice?" These questions direct the co-adventurer's attention to the benefits of the outdoor experience and linking them to life outside the counseling interaction. If what they describe during the session comes to fruition at home, they are more likely to notice it and remember to let you know at your next meeting.

The Tomorrow Question

Otherwise known as the miracle question this is a specific use of "suppose" which is bound to a time and place. "You go to sleep tonight and when you wake in the morning all the challenges bringing you here no longer exist.

What would be the very first thing, the very first and smallest thing, you would notice that told you this was so?" This tool takes us directly to our client's preferred future and helps us construct together a perfect, near perfect, or a good enough day. We grow the client's description from their very first observations to the first person they would see and what they would notice that told them our client was no longer with their "problem."

Because this question may be asked at the start of a multi-day expedition or four-hour session, we must link it to not only the participant's metaphorical *tomorrow*, but our work together. Practitioners can ask what they will notice from their co-adventurers during their outdoor therapy work to indicate they are heading towards their good-enough tomorrow. One technique is to imagine that the client's response to the "tomorrow question" is the last chapter of your work together. What is the chapter that precedes it, and what would the next chapter be from right now? For example, if a co-adventurer mentions wanting to remain clean and sober, we may ask what would happen before reaching that time, and what would be the signs they are heading in that direction.

Getting Stuck

Impasses and treatment failures occur. Most people who engage in our services have previous therapy experiences. They are no stranger to the therapist's couch. Despite delivering our services outdoors, the issues contributing to a lack of progress are the same. Duncan et al.'s (1997) work with therapy veterans is particularly illuminating, as they argued that 1) *anticipating failure*; 2) *discrepancy in theories*; 3) *doing more of what is not working*; and 4) *not taking client motivation into account* are the leading causes of getting stuck.

When we work with people who have long rap sheets, thick case folders, or grave diagnoses, we can anticipate failure. We cite the Rosenhan (1973) experiment which placed perfectly well-adjusted, psychologically sane people into mental institutions in the United States. Despite exhibiting no symptoms of psychosis, they were treated similarly to the other patients, and prescribed antipsychotic medications. Though none of the hospital staff knew it, the "pseudopatients" were flushing their medications down the toilet. All but one were diagnosed with schizophrenia that was in remission prior to their release from the hospital. We are unlikely to explore a person's strengths and resources or elicit hope if we anticipate failure.

One issue with viewing our model of therapy as our best hammer is the tendency to want everything nailed down. We elicit systematic feedback to minimize any discrepancies in theory or our relationship as much as possible.

Co-adventurers should feel safe to tell us when our strategy is off base, thus, we can avoid doing more of what is not working. As stated previously, unmotivated clients do not exist. If we ignore their motivation, they may feel invalidated, as if we did not care to ask what brought them through the door. We should keep Duncan et al.'s (1997) work in mind, as these factors likely contribute to a lack of progress in therapy and issues in the therapeutic alliance. We dive deeper into what we can do with feedback from co-adventurers throughout this book and specifically in Chapter 9. If there is one take away, it is that the practitioner is responsible for a lack of client engagement. We do not want to remove ourselves from the therapeutic relationship by assigning blame for treatment failures on the client.

Conclusion

While the tools described in this chapter may seem easy to incorporate into your practice, we urge practitioners to focus on the assumptions they bring to their work. Reflect on those you work with and how you view presenting problems or stuck cases. Consider how these classic solution-focused tools can be adapted for outdoor use. Outdoor therapy is characterized based on the intentional use of outdoor settings and active bodily engagement (Harper & Dobud, 2020). We described in this chapter the tools we use to process and reflect on the experiences of our co-adventurers. Meaning is constructed through the interaction between practitioner, client, and the outdoor experience. The questions we ask simply bridge the therapy experience to life when the problems bringing that person to therapy are no longer present.

References

American Psychiatric Association [APA]. (2013). Anxiety disorders. In American Psychiatric Association (Ed.), *Diagnostic and statistical manual of mental disorders* (5th ed.) American Psychiatric Association. https://doi.org/10.1176/appi. books.9780890425596.dsm05

Australian Association for Bush Adventure Therapy, Inc. [AABAT]. (2021). *About AABAT*. Retrieved from https://aabat.org.au/about-aabat/

Bannink, F. (2010). *1001 solution-focused questions: Handbook for solution-focused interviewing*. W. W. Norton & Co.

Bliss, E. V., & Bray, D. (2009). The smallest solution focused particles: Towards a minimalist definition of when therapy is solution focused. *Journal of Systemic Therapies*, 28(2), 62–74. https://doi.org/10.1521/jsyt.2009.28.2.62

Clark, J. P., Marmol, L. M., Cooley, R., & Gathercoal, K. (2004). The effects of wilderness therapy on the clinical concerns (on Axes I, II, and IV) of troubled adolescents. *Journal of Experiential Education, 27*(2), 213–232. https://doi.org/10.1177%2F105382590402700207

de Shazer, S. (1989). Resistance revisited. *Contemporary Family Therapy, 11*(4), 227–233. https://doi.org/10.1007/BF00919462

Dobud, W. W. (2020). *Experiences of adventure therapy: A narrative inquiry* [Doctoral Dissertation]. Charles Sturt University.

Dobud, W. W., & Cavanaugh, D. L. (2020). Future direction for outdoor therapies. In N. J. Harper & W. W. Dobud (Eds.), *Outdoor therapies: An introduction to practices, possibilities, and critical perspectives* (pp. 188–202). Routledge.

Dobud, W. W., & Harper, N. J. (2018). Of dodo birds and common factors: A scoping review of direct comparison trials in adventure therapy. *Complementary Therapies in Clinical Practice, 31*, 16–24. https://doi.org/10.1016/j.ctcp.2018.01.005

Duncan, B. L., Hubble, M. A., & Miller, S. D. (1997). *Psychotherapy with "impossible" cases: The efficient treatment of therapy veterans.* WW Norton & Co.

Frank, J. D., & Frank, J. B. (1991). *Persuasion and healing: A comparative study of psychotherapy.* JHU Press.

George, E., Iveson, C., & Ratner, H. (1990). *Problem to solution: Brief therapy with individuals and families.* BT Press.

Goddard, K. (1996). In defence of the past: A response to Ron Wilgosh counselling. In S. Palmer, S. Dainow, & P. Milner (Eds.), *The BAC counselling reader.* SAGE.

Harper, N. J., & Dobud, W. W. (Eds.) (2020). *Outdoor Therapies: An introduction to practices, possibilities, and critical perspectives.* Routledge.

Harper, N. J., Rose, K., & Segal, D. (2019). *Nature-based therapy: A practitioner's guide to working outdoors with children, youth, and families.* New Society Publishers.

Hill, N. R. (2007). Wilderness therapy as a treatment modality for at-risk youth: A primer for mental health counselors. *Journal of Mental Health Counseling, 29*(4), 338–349. https://doi.org/10.17744/mehc.29.4.c6121j162j143178

Kazdin, A. E. (2000). *Encyclopedia of psychology* (Vol. 2). American Psychological Association.

Kelley, S. D., Bickman, L., & Norwood, E. (2010). Evidence-based treatments and common factors in youth psychotherapy. In B. L. Duncan, S. D. Miller, B. E. Wampold, & M. A. Hubble (Eds.), *The heart and soul of change: Delivering what works in therapy* (pp. 325–355). American Psychological Association. https://doi.org/10.1037/12075-011

Krauss, S. E. (2005). Research paradigms and meaning making: A primer. *The Qualitative Report*, 10(4), 758–770. https://doi.org/10.46743/2160-3715/2005.1831

Lew, A., & Bettern, B. L. (1996). *A parent's guide to understanding and motivating children*. Connexions Press.

McKergow, M. (2021). *The next generation of solution focused practice: Stretching the world for new opportunities and progress*. Routledge.

Miller, G., & de Shazer, S. (2000). Emotions in solution-focused therapy: A re-examination. *Family Process*, 39(1), 5–23. https://doi.org/10.1111/j.1545-5300.2000.39103.x

Miller, S. D., Hubble, M. A., Chow, D. L., & Seidel, J. A. (2013). The outcome of psychotherapy: Yesterday, today, and tomorrow. *Psychotherapy*, 50(1), 88–97. https://doi.org/10.1037/a0031097

Misheva, E. (2020). Neuromyths, neurobabble and pseudoscience: The complex relationship between the neuro-disciplines and education. *Child Neuropsychology in Practice* (pp. 9–27). Palgrave Macmillan. https://doi.org/10.1007/978-3-030-64930-2_2

Naor, L., & Mayseless, O. (2021). Therapeutic factors in nature-based therapies: Unraveling the therapeutic benefits of integrating nature in psychotherapy. *Psychotherapy*, 58(4), 576–590. https://doi.org/10.1037/pst0000396

Nature. (2021). End the neglect of young people's mental health. *The International Journal of Science*, 598, 235–236.

Natynczuk, S. (2021). Co-adventuring for change: A solution-focused framework for "unspoken" therapy outdoors. *Relational Child and Youth Care Practice*, 34(4), 58–66.

Natynczuk, S., & Dobud, W. W. (2021). Leave no trace, willful unknowing, and implications from the ethics of sustainability for solution-focused practice outdoors. *Journal of Solution Focused Practices*, 5(2), 7.

Norcross, J. C., & Lambert, M. J. (2011). Psychotherapy relationships that work II. *Psychotherapy*, 48(1), 4–8. https://doi.org/10.1037/a0022180

Nylund, D., & Corsiglia, V. (1994). Becoming solution-focused forced in brief therapy: Remembering something important we already knew. *Journal of Systemic Therapies*, 13(1), 5–12. https://doi.org/10.1521/jsyt.1994.13.1.5

Outdoor Behavioral Healthcare Center [OBH]. (2021). *Outdoor behavioral healthcare center*. Retrieved from www.obhcenter.org/

Peeters, L., & Ringer, M. (2020). Experiential facilitation in the outdoors. In N. J. Harper & W. W. Dobud (Eds.), *Outdoor therapies: An introduction to practices, possibilities, and critical perspectives* (pp. 16–29). Routledge.

Polkinghorne, D. E. (1992). Research methodology in humanistic psychology. *The Humanistic Psychologist, 20*(2–3), 218–242. https://doi.org/10.1080/08873267.19 92.9986792

Ratner, H., George, E., & Iveson, C. (2012). *Solution focused brief therapy: 100 key points and techniques*. Routledge.

Rogers, C. R. (1980). *A way of being*. Houghton Mifflin Harcourt.

Rosenhan, D. L. (1973). On being sane in insane places. *Science, 179*(4070), 250–258. https://doi.org/10.1126/science.179.4070.250

Selekman, M. D. (2005). *Pathways to change: Brief therapy with difficult adolescents* (2nd ed.) Guilford Publishing.

Shennan, G. (2019). Acknowledgement and possibility: Coping questions and more. In G. Shennan (Ed.), *Solution-focused practice: Effective communication to facilitate change* (2nd ed.) (Chapter 7). Red Globe Press. http://dx.doi.org/10.1007/978-1-137-31633-2_7

Smith, J. K. (1983). Quantitative versus qualitative research: An attempt to clarify the issue. *Educational Researcher, 12*(3), 6–13. https://doi.org/10.3102%2F00131 89X012003006

Sparks, J., Duncan, B. L., & Miller, S. D. (2007). Common factors and the uncommon heroism of youth. *Psychotherapy in Australia, 13*(2), 34–43.

Substance Abuse and Mental Health Services Administration [SAMHSA]. (2021). *SAMHSA – Substance Abuse and Mental Health Services Administration*. Retrieved from www.samhsa.gov/

Thomas, F. N. (2007). Possible limitations, misunderstandings, and misuses of solution-focused brief therapy. In T. Nelson & F. N. Thomas (Eds.), *Handbook of solution-focused brief therapy: Clinical applications* (pp. 404–421). The Haworth Press.

Wampold, B. E., & Imel, Z. E. (2015). *The great psychotherapy debate: The evidence for what makes psychotherapy work* (2nd ed.). Routledge.

Wettersten, K. B., Lichtenberg, J. W., & Mallinckrodt, B. (2005). Associations between working alliance and outcome in solution-focused brief therapy and brief interpersonal therapy. *Psychotherapy Research, 15*(1–2), 35–43. https://doi.org/10.1080/10503300512331327029

Yusuf, D. (Ed.) (2021). *The solution focused approach with children and young people: Current thinking and practice*. Routledge.

Part II
Outdoor Solution-Focused Practice

4
Being Solution-Focused Outdoors

"...it is better to travel hopefully than to arrive..."
Robert Louis Stevenson (1881, p. 190)

No matter the experience or theoretical orientation, listening is a good place to start. Then practitioners can develop skills in applying Carl Rogers' (1957) core conditions of change, which include congruence, unconditional positive regard, confidentiality, and empathy, as perceived by the participant. Egan's (2002) *Skilled Helper* model, which is broadly integrative and pragmatic rather than theoretically dogmatic or diagnostic, seems a useful initial approach for non-professional counselors. Qualifying as an accredited psychotherapist takes years, requiring further education, money, training, and hundreds of hours of clinically supervised practice. An important consideration is to decide which therapeutic modality you are the most philosophically aligned with, as you will have to practice with conviction and authenticity.

No matter your qualification or level of training and experience, we use this chapter to link solution-focused practice to relevant ideas for outdoor practice. Outdoor therapy practitioners require a balancing of psychotherapy skills and outdoor facilitation. First, we present host leadership as a framework for outdoor therapy practice and inquire about the importance of success and mastery. We then examine our concerns with viewing experience as technique. What follows is a look at the Disneyfication of outdoor pursuits, and an exploration of risk management and ethical considerations for this work.

Host Leadership

The back cover of Mark McKergow's and Pierluigi Pugliese's (2019) *Field Manual* reads "Leading as a host is about bringing people together to address

DOI: 10.4324/9781003217558-6

complex collective problems." From first hearing Mark talk of host leadership, I (Stephan) knew this was one of those things I wish I thought up myself. One of the main attractions of this model was in the reframing of clients, not as customers, though as guests. The model applies itself well to adventurous journeying, whether a four-hour cave trip or a multi-day expedition, and I have written about host leadership in adventure therapy in detail elsewhere (Natynczuk, 2019). The host leadership model has its roots in solution-focused practice and a typical introductory description of the model invites one to consider hosting a dinner party.

The host deliberately invites people who would contribute to an enjoyable social time around a good meal. The invitation is specific in bringing people together who have something in common, who might get along in social situations and will entertain each other, and perhaps make new connections. The host meets guests at the door, politely welcomes them in, ensures their comfort, offers a drink and some nibbles. They introduce each newly arrived guest to the others, perhaps mentioning something they have in common to ease this newly expanded group into conversation. As the night goes on, the host moves to the kitchen to replenish a plate of canapés, open another bottle, or check the oven, and returns to the group to ensure no-one is feeling left out. Should someone's presence become inappropriate, the host might politely ask that guest to take time out, leave, or call for a taxi.

For our role in working outdoors, practitioners carefully select their guests – we might call them clients, or co-adventurers – with a purpose in mind common to all other members of the group, including ourselves as we take part in the shared adventure as co-facilitators of change. We know to be flexible, to listen, and build on each answer as we move together towards a solution. That flexibility is important in our complex role as leader, guide, instructor, and therapist. A wrong move and the therapeutic relationship can be ruptured to the point where leadership is in doubt and any therapeutic efficacy is lost. There may be times when we need to be didactic, to temporarily be the hero-type leader, perhaps in a rescue where our technical experience, knowledge, and training come into urgent play. As host leaders, we can do these things as the model is flexible and overarching on any spectrum of leadership styles. However, it is important to discuss with the group what leadership looks like early on so there are no surprises when things need to change.

The host performs several leadership roles: *Initiator, Inviter, Space Creator, Gatekeeper, Co-Participator,* and *Connector.* Table 4.1 illustrates how these roles translate to the outdoor therapy scenario. Appendix F in the field manual provides space for practitioners to reflect on the strengths and areas in

Table 4.1 Host Leadership Roles in Outdoor Therapy

	Role	Considerations for Outdoor Therapy
In Preparation	Initiator	Prior to hosting any experience, practitioners reflect on their passion to pursue outdoor therapy. They ask, "What makes this a good idea?" They consider the guest list and what they will need in order to facilitate a meaningful experience. This includes outdoor equipment, certificates, permissions, and considerations about the outdoor setting, taking into account weather and risk management.
	Inviter	Reflect on the perfect co-adventurer(s) for the experience. How could the outdoor therapy experience benefit them? Practitioners make sure to define the desired outcome, not necessarily the process. Offer the choice for participants to accept or decline the invitation. It is useful to communicate a sense of warmth and acceptance when inviting people to your outdoor therapy experience. Practitioners communicate that participants' attendance matters. Remaining invitational is at the heart of host leadership. Participants are provided information about what to expect from their attendance, so as not to be caught off guard.
	Space Creator	At a dinner party, creating space could relate to what music is chosen to play in the background and when the food is served. Similar considerations are needed for outdoor therapy. Practitioners take time to consider meal choices, the outdoor equipment provided, and how they schedule the experience altogether. Outdoor settings are kept clean and organized during the experience. Practitioners offer to clean any mess or repair damaged equipment. Considerations are made for what the appearance of the practitioner and the outdoor setting communicate to the co-adventurer(s).

(Continued)

Table 4.1 Host Leadership Roles in Outdoor Therapy (*Cont'd*)

	Role	Considerations for Outdoor Therapy
During the Experience	Gatekeeper	Now that the experience has started, practitioners are at the threshold of inviting people through the door. Boundaries and agreements are contracted with the co-adventurer(s). These boundaries are not too rigid and invite consensus on what will lead to group safety. They make decisions about what should be encouraged or discouraged. The outdoor therapy practitioner observes the group to handle anything that arises. If something is going awry, the practitioner steps in to ensure safety and improve client engagement.
	Connector	Outdoor therapy practitioners are familiar with the pros and cons of facilitating ice breaker activities to help participants get to know each other. Practitioners ensure no one is left out and that the group is seamlessly transitioning to the next phase of the experience, such as a meal around the fire during an expedition. Practitioners may provide ideas for conversation or invite the group members to get to know each other on their own, avoiding being the center of attention. They remain aware that sometimes they can leave their co-adventurer(s) to simply get on with it and wait for possibilities to occur.
	Co-Participator	Though practitioners host the experience, they eventually join in and participate with the co-adventurer(s). They share meals together, use similar outdoor equipment, take part in all activities, and join during informal conversations. They step back to allow the co-adventurer(s) to eat first and monitor their experience of comfort and safety in the outdoor setting.

need of development based on these leadership roles. Building on the dinner party metaphor, we *invite* participants to an outdoor *space* and *co-participate* in outdoor activities together. We *connect* participants with others in group settings and *initiate* discussions about people's preferred future.

Everyone in attendance is deliberately chosen for a particular event and contributes to the successful interaction. It is the deliberate invitation that initially distinguishes this leadership model. This builds on the *Servant Leader* framework (Greenleaf, 1970), where the leader facilitates a group process in the background, builds community with a purpose, and quietly ensures everything is in place for success.

There are four positions of the host leader: *in the spotlight, with the guests, in the gallery*, and *in the kitchen* (McKergow & Bailey, 2014). Outdoor therapy practitioners may be in the spotlight when teaching a skill or describing the landscape. Additionally, there might be times when practitioners must intervene in order to keep participants safe. They might facilitate discussion, facilitate an activity, or ask solution-focused questions to establish meaningful dialogue.

With the theme of co-adventuring, practitioners spend much of their time with their guests. Research suggests outdoor therapy recipients prefer to see the human side of their practitioners and prefer the establishing of a *real relationship* (Gelso et al., 2018). Practitioners spend time informally building relationships with co-adventurers. They remember important information about those they interact with, such as the names of their pets or what position they play in football.

Experienced outdoor facilitators will be used to the gallery. This position takes place at a distance, where practitioners can survey the participants. They take a pause from all the business and observe the group interaction, and keep an eye on safety. Practitioners reflect on the challenges ahead and consider what changes they could make when they step back into the spotlight. In expedition settings, the group of practitioners can step away during an activity and observe how the group of participants functions together. They may also process what has occurred during the day when everyone else is asleep.

The final position of the host leader is in the kitchen. Back to the dinner party metaphor again, the host may retreat to the kitchen to take a deep breath and gather themselves. Co-workers may join you in the kitchen, but the guests are usually steered towards other places. Practitioners use the "kitchen" to reflect on their work, to take time out, or engage in clinical supervision or coaching. We encourage practitioners to schedule their time in the kitchen, especially to reduce the risk of burnout or exhaustion.

There is one function of host leadership not getting much mention in the literature, and that is how to wrap things up at the end of the dinner party or to close an expedition. We know endings are important in therapy, and they should be managed. As solution-focused practitioners we immediately start work with the ending in mind. How we manage the end of a therapeutic adventure demands some sensitive consideration. How do we say goodbye? How do we deal with the bonds developed during such meaningful time together? Are the roles of Gatekeeper and Connector still important at the end of the work? Is it just a matter of counting down to the time to depart as we might during an indoor therapy session? Debriefing, summarizing, appreciating, and affirming might be some of the important things to do at the completion of the venture. Leadership does not stop as soon as everyone has gone home. In the dinner party analogy, there is still the tidying up to do, the washing up, emptying the bins, and the gathering of lost property.

Host leadership is a guiding principle to this approach of solution-focused practice in outdoor therapy. The metaphors fit seamlessly. Practitioners are reminded that their work involves facilitating, and hosting, an "experience." The purpose of the relationship is to facilitate experiences of success and mastery. If you work with someone certain that therapy is destined for failure, your relationship could be the co-adventurer's first sign of hope. Next comes success and mastery, which we visit below.

Reconceptualizing Success and Mastery

Success and mastery are not terms reserved for outdoor facilitation. They have been used in psychotherapy literature for decades (Frank & Frank, 1991). The Outward Bound model presented by Walsh and Golins (1976) demonstrated how experiences of success and mastery can be one pathway for change. Frank and Frank (1991) suggested: "Performances attributed to their own efforts enhance self-esteem more strongly than those they attribute to such external factors as medication or outside help" (p. 49). If participants arrive to us reporting levels of subjective wellbeing well below clinical cutoffs (DeMille et al., 2018), experiences of self-efficacy could elicit a participant's self-empowerment for problem solving.

Some may experience success through talking, such as when building insight about a past experience of overcoming the urge to self-harm. Others may benefit from a more active behavioral experience, like mastering the J or C stroke while paddling from the stern of a canoe. Frank and Frank (1991) described that in its heyday, certain schools of psychotherapy, such as psychodynamic practitioners, believed suffering to be the cause of emotional blocks, or defenses, and were due to a person's parental upbringing. For those with neurological and intellectual developmental concerns, this insight-oriented therapy left people more demoralized than when they arrived. The basic assumption here was that for these people to change, they must understand the degree to which their problems impacted their lives and accept the responsibility for the situation. In our practice, we focus firsthand on facilitating experiences of success and mastery, no matter one's actual abilities. Success and mastery depend on "whether it exceeds or falls below the person's expectations" (p. 49).

Consider the case vignette shared by Karoff et al. (2017) about implementing adventure therapy into a peer-to-peer support program for adolescents diagnosed with autism spectrum disorder. The authors described a student named Adam, who struggled socially. He avoided eye contact with his peers, would walk the halls looking at the ground, and disengage when frustrated. Throughout the program, Adam "gained consistent practice in social interactions, first through participation when invited to engage, and then gradually becoming more comfortable with initiating interaction" (p. 402). When Adam preferred to isolate, he was still invited to be the group's timekeeper. Interpreted through our reconceptualization of success and mastery, this may have been the perfect tailoring, based on Adam's capabilities, for him to achieve this pathway for change.

Success, and mastery in particular, are not just nice things to add on to your outdoor therapeutic work so your clients "feel better." Mastery elicits hope (Frank & Frank, 1991). Remember, many people strapping on their boots to join us for a nature walk may not be too hopeful that therapy works. However, if during that experience they feel a sense of natural mindfulness, or successfully cross a stream jumping from rock to rock, or feel a sense of group cohesion, they may sense they are in the right place.

In Chapter 2, we examined Howard et al.' (1986, 1993, 1996) work on how much therapy is required before we should expect change to occur. Despite arguments about long- or short-term interventions, most therapy recipients tend to experience change at a similar rate: sooner rather than later. The longer we work with someone reporting no benefit, the less likely benefit is to come. It is tempting to attribute the lack of progress to trauma, stigma, or resistance. Success and mastery, and the therapeutic alliance, are useful factors to consider with stuck cases. For the remainder of this section, we revisit Walsh and Golins' (1976) work to take another look at success and mastery, our aim being to develop this tool for practitioners to consider when approaching their work.

Walsh and Golins (1976) wrote it "is rewarding to master OUTWARD BOUND because it presents the kinds of problems the human being is de-signed to solve" (p. 13). The authors argued the cognitive, affective, and psychomotor ingredients of programs, or thinking, emotions, and physical taxonomies, are present to complement one's ability to resolve problems. The process they outline describes how to "reorganize" someone's abilities to solve problems. This is not language we would use to describe our work, though we do urge practitioners to reconsider how important this model is for conceptualizing outdoor therapy. Below, we have outlined how this was written in 1976, followed by our musings on how to use such theory in solution-focused practice outdoors:

> They are presented the problem (receiving), (perception), and (knowledge). They then translate the problem into their own lan-guage (comprehension), accept the problem (respond), and prepare to solve it (preparating). In doing the latter they might gather around one another to confer, cinch up their belts, etc. Having applied or seen the application of various bodily configurations before (appli-cation), they begin to plan by analyzing all the variables involved (analysis), to initiate the plans with a set of values (valuing – it may be to solve the problem honestly without the use of gimmicks), and they begin to act out various options physically (orientation). Some may test the wall, some may lift others to ascertain strengths, etc. Then they decide on a plan (synthesis), follow through on it (organization), and put it into action (pattern). Finally, they are totally involved and committed to its execution (performance and characterization), and as they master the task they inevitably (evaluate) it, (their plan either succeeds or it does not).
>
> (pp. 13–14)

This is clearly a mouthful. When a co-adventurer experiences success and mastery, the solution-focused practitioner asks useful questions about what difference the experience can make in the person's future. Just as we aim to construct a climate of competence, the outdoor experiences we share are focused on facilitating this sense of mastery. The successful accomplishment of certain initiatives becomes the exception to the very problems bringing people to therapy.

Naomi, 24 years old, was referred to a government-funded seven-day outdoor therapy expedition. She was born in a regional area and suffered from fetal alcohol spectrum disorder. Her adoptive parents were concerned by the lack of job prospects and motivation to pursue any social life outside of substance using in the community. Naomi was visibly angry during the first hike, which was facilitated by a social worker and outdoor guide. The practitioners stopped the hike and validated her frustration. Instead of hiking with the backpack, the three co-adventurers agreed to set up a base camp and go for day hikes each day. She would not have to carry the heavy backpack. Naomi enjoyed watching the wildlife, especially the birds, and practiced reading a book to learn their names. On day three, Naomi proclaimed, "See! I can do it!" as she reached the top of the mountain. "Amazing!" the social worker responded. "How were you able to do that?" Naomi mentioned that she sometimes forgets how strong she really is. This became a theme during the remainder of the expedition. Naomi's parents called the organization a week after the experience to report that Naomi had landed a job as a cleaner in a restaurant. During a follow-up phone call, Naomi told the two practitioners that she knew she was smart from knowing the names of so many birds and treated the job interview like hiking the mountain.

The practitioners in this story were mindful that co-constructing success and mastery was essential to increasing therapeutic value. When Naomi hated the hiking, they paused and carefully crafted alternatives – as a good host will do when someone arrives with a dietary requirement. They found exceptions to the problem, which Naomi's mother described as a lack of engagement in any education or future. When Naomi wanted to learn about birds, the practitioners followed. It was a slow process as Naomi read at a third grade reading level. When Naomi exhibited what appeared to be success and mastery, whether through correctly identifying wildlife or scaling the mountain, the practitioners asked questions that helped Naomi know the mastery occurred because of her own doing. The practitioners appropriated no change to themselves, despite hosting what would become a meaningful experience.

Success and mastery, as perceived by the co-adventurer, is one pathway for change. A strong therapeutic relationship is another (Norcross & Lambert, 2011). When we focus on our specific techniques and the particulars of our interventions, we risk losing sight of these two key predictors of change. Along with the concerns of viewing experience as technique, we present in the following section how we can treat co-adventurers with *fierce dignity* (Pringle et al., 2021).

Experiential as Technique

We are frequently asked what activities outdoor facilitators should use to construct therapeutic meaning. The tendency here is to focus on activities. Just like seasoned psychotherapists, techniques, activities, and cleverly manufactured acronyms have a seductive allure. In group supervision, we have heard, "Who has a good activity for social anxiety?" While it is useful to add more strategies to your outdoor therapy toolkit, you risk becoming problem-focused, and diagnostic, by adopting techniques designed for specific symptomatic criteria, and the therapy can be lost. At a supervision session for practitioners some years ago, I (Stephan) recall listening to accounts of activities for diagnoses and asking "Where is the therapy?" and this brought the session to a juddering halt. Context matters, and any description of psychotherapy void of contextual factors risks becoming solution-*forced*.

Outdoor facilitators from all backgrounds and training may run into therapeutic groups and may not have a lot of time with their co-adventurers. For instance, consider taking groups to high ropes courses, where the majority of processing is delivered by the ropes course staff. When we do not have a lot of time with a group, it becomes more important to allow space for meaning to be constructed by the participants. The best ideas for change come from the person aiming to make said change.

For example, before doing a blindfolded climb up a telephone pole, the ropes course facilitator says, "This is a great activity to work on your communication skills." The facilitator is prescribing their own meaning and value to the experience. Sure, a participant may finish the climb and mention how important open communication is, though if we do not prescribe meaning, they may experience trust, faith, or any other meaning they have made. Activities hold no inherent meaning or value until co-adventurers experience them. In true solution-focused manner, we are not experts in how people experience our work. We ask useful questions to evoke meaning. Meaning freely constructed from experience is most powerful.

This may look like a small hill for us to die on, but outdoor experiential facilitation is vulnerable to a "techno-rational framework" (Roberts, 2005, p. 16). The more restricted the activities we facilitate, the more we limit *experience*. When using words like *experiential*, we must not disregard their philosophical underpinnings. Roberts (2005) argued that moving from "experience" to "experiential" has a dark side where we can lose the democratic environment early experiential facilitators, like John Dewey, argued for all along. We tend to "see experience through a techno-rational lens, as an isolated activity, or technique, to achieve specified and prescribed objectives" (p. 22).

We remind our readers of the Dodo Bird's verdict presented in Chapter 2. Though outdoor therapy scholars have long questioned what *active ingredients* contribute to client outcomes, such as hiking, group interaction, or time outdoors, we have little evidence that these factors are required or necessary. If we removed one particular activity from a wilderness therapy program, one that the staff and clinical directors view is essential, what would happen? Would outcomes actually decline? It is hard to say, but research from our neighboring psychotherapies is telling. For example, in dismantling studies of eye movement desensitization and reprocessing, a therapy designed for the treatment of trauma, identical outcomes are achieved without any eye movements at all, bringing us to question the very technique the therapy was named after. Dismantling outdoor therapies, while called for in the literature (Dobud & Harper, 2018), has yet to be conducted, and you can try this yourself.

For an interesting critical reflection, you might journal on the factors you think most likely to contribute to change. List the activities you find central to your programming. If you are on expedition, do you require your co-adventurers to journal? Are they allowed to bring a mobile phone? Workers experienced in overnight programming bring many assumptions about what is most important. However, we must remain mindful that the techniques and activities themselves, and many of our assumptions about the efficacy of our practice frameworks, have little evidence to support their impact in isolation to the context of our relationships, a co-adventurer's motivation, and how these activities are, in fact, *experienced*.

Solution-focused questioning can evoke information about what your client took away from the experience and help to consolidate gains made during the activity. Listen for change talk from participants and be aware of body language. Was the supposedly distractible child able to remain focused while navigating with a map and compass? If so, inquire about it. The map and compass did not help the child improve their attention, they did it themselves, *through* the experience set in a meaningful context. The practitioner helps to build meaning on the experience through the line of inquiry. The map and compass hold no inherent value, and when a co-adventurer shows little interest in the endeavor, we ditch it.

McDonalds and the Disneyfication of Outdoor Experiences

"Do you want fries with that?" wrote Jay W. Roberts (2005, p. 19) in his article "Disney, Dewey, and the Death of Experience in Education." The concept of McDonaldization relates to the adoption of a fast-food restaurant mindset when it comes to education, travel, healthcare, and politics. For Ritzer (1996), the four dimensions of McDonaldization are: 1) efficacy; 2) calculability; 3) predictability; and 4) control. You can see this occurring in pursuits for recognition for evidence-based status on various databases, such as the SAMHSA's (2021) *National Registry for Evidence-Based Programs and Practices*. Context and relationships are veiled to mechanistic views of change. The medical model pokes its head out again.

What happens when McDonaldization trumps *experience* can be problematic. Practitioners become process-oriented (Duncan et al., 2004). Focusing on process, they fixate on why their work is not more broadly recognized. A noble pursuit, for sure, but one that can lead to a lot of unjustified hype. Certain approaches are manualized in an attempt to make all therapy taste the same. As Roberts (2005) argued, the Big Mac in New York better taste the same as the one in Los Angeles. A wilderness therapy program in Utah better look similar to one in North Carolina. The aim is to remove the human component; hence it is no surprise many researchers describe the variance in individual therapists as a *nuisance variable* (Miller et al., 2013). To McDonaldize outdoor therapy is another reason why referring to co-adventurers as consumers, customers, or service users is problematic (Loynes, 1998). Some argue this stance is arbitrary, though making this all the more frightening is the Western world's preference for manualized therapies, which despite the efforts from all the king's horses, researchers, and advocates alike have not been able to quell those ever inconvenient wild cards: therapists and clients (Wampold & Imel, 2015).

Experience gets watered down when we focus on process. A school principal might call and ask if you can do some team-building activities with their 8th grade students. "Same price as usual right?" she asks. We do not wish to come across as naive here. This is how much of the Western world operates. We compete against each other for funding and create turf battles about whose techniques are better. However, the delivery of canned outdoor experiences, whether therapeutic, educational, or recreational, is worrying.

In Chapter 3, we presented the questions we may ask co-adventurers. We stressed that when we pretend that we know what answers someone will give us, we will feel surprised and rattled about what to do next if their answers differ. Additionally, if a client does not fit into how we want them to act, learn, or grow, we risk treating them as resistant to our practice. If we ignore people's strengths, resources, and capabilities, we may adopt the Killer D's (Duncan, 2014) we discussed in Chapter 1, inflating the contributions of the practitioner, thus reducing opportunities for self-determination, and getting stuck instead of moving on in the work.

Dignity of Risk

The term *dignity of risk* came from pastoral counselor Robert Perske (1972), an advocate for the rights of people with mental health concerns. At the time, people diagnosed with intellectual disabilities were considered to be incapable of independent living, an assumption depriving many of opportunities to experience what most of us would consider to be typical life events, such as intimate relationships, the right to choose what food to eat, and the ability to experience the same risks as the general public. Perske's (1972) conceptualization has been appropriated to aged care and outdoor education, but its discussion has been limited in the outdoor therapies. In this section, we explore dignity of risk when taking therapy outdoors and link this discussion to self-determination and care.

When people are institutionalized, such as those placed in aged care, the practitioners involved can do all they can to minimize all risks in order to keep their clients safe. For example, an 80-year-old male might want to walk to the local supermarket, but staff view him as frail and unable to navigate the nearby intersection. Despite elevated cholesterol or risk of type-2 diabetes, someone may wish to drink a soft drink each day with their lunch, followed by a sticky date pudding. All of these scenarios include risk, and the elderly are certainly more vulnerable than the general public. However, removing these opportunities due to the potential risk may diminish experiences for self-determination, autonomy, and the human right to experience. According to Perske (1972):

> Overprotection may appear on the surface to be kind, but it can be really evil. An oversupply can smother people emotionally, squeeze the life out of their hopes and expectations, and strip them of their dignity. Overprotection can keep people from becoming all they could become. Many of our best achievements came the hard way: We took risks, fell flat, suffered, picked ourselves up, and tried again. Sometimes we made it and sometimes we did not. Even so, we were given the chance to try. Persons with special needs need these chances, too. Of course, we are talking about prudent risks. People should not be expected to

blindly face challenges that, without a doubt, will explode in their faces. Knowing which chances are prudent and which are not – this is a new skill that needs to be acquired. On the other hand, a risk is really only when it is not known beforehand whether a person can succeed. The real world is not always safe, secure, and predictable, it does not always say "please," "excuse me," or "I'm sorry." Every day we face the possibility of being thrown into situations where we will have to risk everything… In the past, we found clever ways to build avoidance of risk into the lives of persons living with disabilities. Now we must work equally hard to help find the proper amount of risk these people have the right to take. We have learned that there can be healthy development in risk taking and there can be crippling indignity in safety!

(n.p.)

Writing a risk management plan is important for any hazardous scenario, but it can quickly become a nuisance. In one workplace, we reviewed one organization's policies and noticed a *shark attack prevention* plan. The policy ordered adventure guides to prevent any participant from going knee deep in the ocean, despite the expedition taking place in a coastal environment during the early summer. It was hot and humid. Participants requested going in the water to cool down, but we were instructed to police such risky behavior due to the off chance of a great white shark attack.

Obviously, a bizarre example, though we have heard about other policies which may impact a co-adventurer's dignity. For example, participants in many US wilderness therapy programs are told to yell their name or the number designated to them repeatedly whenever out of staff's earshot, including when toileting (Dobud, 2020). They are instructed never to speak with one another if a staff member cannot hear their conversation. Their shoes are taken each night, as well as their belts or any rope, to prevent runaway or self-harm. Men and women alike have no access to razors for shaving, effectively withholding people's choice to treat their body how they wish (Mitten, 1994). While these are brash responses to previous negative wilderness therapy experiences, the impact these have on someone's right to self-determination and dignity are profound, let alone the impact on any useful therapeutic alliance.

We describe in Chapter 6 how we should be mindful about the "rules" we impose on outdoor therapy participants. We can distract them with lists of rules to follow. In fact, some programs we have observed require participants to memorize a list of rules prior to allowing full participation (Dobud, 2021). This is too prescriptive, paternalistic, and coercive to be anything like the solution-focused practice we strive for. These approaches reduce opportunities for clients' creativity and curiosity.

While conducting program observation research in Norway, I (Will) was taken aback by how the interdisciplinary team maintained the co-adventurers' dignity of risk. In fact, I was quite shocked and, honestly, felt uncomfortable based on the training I had received in the United States. On the final night of our program, while sleeping in a small cabin, the participants stayed up all night talking to each other, despite all staff heading off to our respective bunk beds. I never worked for a program that would have allowed such an occurrence. In the morning, the participants appeared exhausted with large rings under their eyes. They had stayed up for the morning sunrise. During our final hike, I asked the participants what they did all night, sure it had to be something sexual or risky. What they did, however, was talk about their plans for enacting their goals, staying connected with each other, and watching the sunrise because, "Time in nature is healing." I was thrilled and stunned. Maybe the way I was trained limited the creativity and curiosity of adolescents by remaining too concerned with risk!

A Note on Ethics

A unified code of ethics is possibly the main hurdle to professionalizing outdoor therapies (Natynczuk, 2016, 2019). Most social workers and counselors who belong to a professional body will have a code of ethics (e.g., Australian Association for Social Workers, 2020) and should it be broken then the practitioner can lose their professional status. Instructors, adventure sport coaches, and guides might have a code of practice to follow that comes with their qualifications and any association they belong to for a particular award, for example the British Caving Association, or the British Canoe Union, though are unlikely to have their awards taken away for anything other than the most grievous misdemeanor. Following a successful prosecution, or even much adverse publicity, practitioners would find it very challenging to secure employment, or private clients, due to such a blow to their reputation. The picture is complicated by jurisdictions placing varying demands on outdoor therapy practitioners: some emphasize regulations on counseling skills and make few demands on practitioners to show qualifications in outdoor recreation, others vice versa.

Ethics are important to professional organizations (Howard, 1996) and to business in general (Caldwell, 2015). Outdoor therapy practitioners are not an exception. Having an ethical code in place demands a disciplinary policy for transgressions, which could lead to expulsion from the professional association (Gray, 2011). Khele et al. (2008) investigated complaints to the

British Association for Counselling and Psychotherapy and found the disciplinary system of a professional association needs the teeth to maintain a good level of credibility. Caldwell (2015) reiterated that most breaches of ethical practice go undisclosed, and when reported, little follow-up occurs. In which case, one might question the point of having an ethical code if it means little or nothing such that practitioners can behave as they wish with no consequences for bad, dangerous, or even illegal practice.

What can we learn from other vocations and professions that overlap with outdoor therapy? Ethical codes for coaching associations are broadly similar (Gray, 2011). The European Mentoring and Coaching Council's (2016) Global Code of Ethics brings practitioners together from diverse practice and over multiple jurisdictions throughout Europe. It may be a good model for an outdoor practitioner's code of practice as it asks practitioners to ensure their competence is a match for their client's needs. Practitioners must understand the context of their work, of conflicts of interest and boundary issues. Confidentiality must be maintained, and they must not exploit clients in any way, even through seeking testimonials (Caldwell, 2015).

There have been a small number of ethical codes and best practice guidelines intended for outdoor therapy practitioners, such as those generated by the Australian Association for Bush Adventure Therapy (2021) and the Association for Experiential Education's Certified Clinical Adventure Therapist scheme (2021). Both are particular to their home nations, Australia and the United States respectively, and illustrate well the challenges of finding a universal ethics code. We feel very strongly that ethics must be rigorous and robust and go far beyond casual opinions of what is right and wrong. Ethics are not inconvenient to what we want to do. They require transparency and practitioners must be honest about owning and adhering to them. Giving ethics the cold shoulder is not to be used as excuses for otherwise unacceptable behavior, especially when measured against such standards as the United Nations Human Rights Convention (1948) and European Convention on Human Rights (1998).

For those tied to a certain profession, such as social work or psychology, we recommend adhering to your governing body's ethics as the absolute foundation to your practice. For example, a qualified social worker is a social worker first, outdoor therapy practitioner second. Dobud's (2020) dissertation focused on experiences of adolescents in outdoor therapy practice. The inquiry found some wilderness therapy programs sticking with aged policies and procedures seemingly at odds of best ethical conduct as stated by the relevant social work code of ethics. In this case, many practitioners seemed to follow their organizational policies, despite being required to adhere to their professional guidelines.

The past few years we thought hard about ethics for outdoor therapy we could borrow from outdoor best practice that worked as a handy metaphor for therapy outdoors (Natynczuk & Dobud, 2021). The ideal of these sustainability ethics to leave no trace on the natural environments we recreate was consistent and familiar to our solution-focused outdoor practice.

Leave No Trace in Your Client's Life

Our interest has always been in the seamless join between therapy and outdoor pursuits, and the blend therein. A vital link seemed to be missing that might define the blend for us. How could we bring the great outdoors and talking therapy together making their union less clunky and relatively effortless? The Leave No Trace (LNT) ethic for sustainability was a perfect fit and we extended our thinking to a discussion of privilege and decolonizing our practice outdoors, which we suggest solution-focused practice lends itself to as long as we are respecting our clients' experience, trusting them to know what they need, and dignifying their answers to our questions designed to help them get the change they want for themselves. Curious readers are directed to our LNT paper, which is easy to find online (Natynczuk & Dobud, 2021).

We have reproduced the summary in Table 4.2 and reproduced Table A.5 in the field manual (Appendix G). The table speaks to the metaphors gained from the LNT principles, their relationship with outdoor practice, therapeutic practice, and solution-focused tools. The principles of LNT include 1) *plan ahead and prepare*; 2) *travel and camp on durable surfaces*; 3) *dispose of waste properly*; 4) *leave what you find*; 5) *minimize campfire impacts*; 6) *respect wildlife*; and 7) *be considerate of other visitors*. At first, readers may struggle to find metaphors relating to their outdoor therapy practice. Taking the second principle to travel on durable surfaces, we made a clear link to focusing on client strengths, resources, resiliencies, and capabilities. We work with what makes our co-adventurers "durable," if you will.

Leaving no trace aligns with Insoo Kim Berg's notion of "leaving no footprints" in our clients' lives. The solution-focused outdoor therapy experience is a moment for the client to be at their best. We avoid retraumatizing people by carelessly wandering through their past. This should not discount

Table 4.2 Principles of Leave No Trace for Solution-Focused Outdoor Therapy

Leave No Trace	Outdoor Practice	General Therapeutic Practice	Solution-Focused Practice
Plan Ahead and Prepare	• Consent and contracting. • Appropriate medical history. • Thorough risk assessment is recommended. • Choice of venue, route, timings, duration, location of facilities, pacing, late return/emergency call-out and communication, local byelaws, access, maps, compass, technical equipment, clothing with regard to climate and weather forecast, spare clothing, head torches, first aid kit, emergency shelter, facility to make a hot drink and so forth.	• Being able to cope with unexpected occurrences takes on a new meaning, especially in unfamiliar environments. • Walk and talk pace can be very slow, the weather has a huge impact. • Terrain has to be appropriate to clients' fitness – it is difficult to talk when out of breath. • Pacing conversation with respect to the effort of moving. • Know places on your route where privacy is easier to find. • For short walks know the route, timings and places you can stand aside from the path while deep contemplation occurs. • There are so many metaphors in the outdoors that can help or hinder. • Understand the importance of landscape and how environment and nature can interact as co-facilitator. • Anticipate the impact of distractions, such as playful dogs and chatty interlopers. • Know how to finish the session if the route outlasts the conversation or vice versa.	• Clients bring their own resources and strengths, both personal and in their social networks. • Prepare to acknowledge the changes occurring all the time. • Regard clients as resourceful and capable of change. • Before the session, think of your client at their best.

| **Travel, Work, and Camp on Durable Surfaces** | • Reduce erosion, soil damage, habitat destruction. | • Stay on the surface, not digging too deep unless it is helpful.
• Do not make assumptions.
• Do not give unsolicited advice. | • Work with your clients' resilience, strengths, and instances of coping well.
• Clients' solutions are more likely to fit their particular situation and are more likely to be implemented and maintained.
• Work with what works well.
• Understand what your client wants from the session.
• Work with your client to navigate to their preferred future, or the destination for the session. |

(Continued)

Table 4.2 Principles of Leave No Trace for Solution-Focused Outdoor Therapy (Cont'd)

Leave No Trace	Outdoor Practice	General Therapeutic Practice	Solution-Focused Practice
Dispose of Waste Properly	• Bag and take away all forms of waste in a hard leakproof container. • Do not pollute water sources. • Do not bury or burn rubbish.	• Take care not to ask careless questions and apologize for the "stupid" questions. • Avoid "diagnosing" your client through the lens of your own experience.	• Avoid countertransference and prescribing "solutions" from one's own narrative and experiences. • The client is the expert.
Leave What You Find	• Do not remove flora, fauna, or artifacts. • Do not add graffiti or carve natural surfaces. • Do not hack at vegetation unnecessarily, or throw rocks recklessly over cliffs or down steep slopes.	• Respect the client's experience and position of expert on themselves. • Maintain confidentiality.	• Respect clients' knowledge and preferences of what they want from talking with you. • Do not be a tourist in clients' lives. • The client is not the problem.

| Minimize Campfire Impacts | • Avoid scorching the ground, take care not to set peat or grassland or forests on fire.
• Use established fire pits, avoid excessive smoke, and keep fires as small as possible.
• If the fire is too big, we do not know what damage we will find should we leave it unattended.
• Extinguish all fires.
• Tidy fire pits and replace turf if digging a fresh pit. | • Avoid re-invoking or causing further trauma.
• Do not dig deep into issues you cannot extinguish before the session's end.
• Avoid insensitivity and insincerity. | • Be careful giving praise, should it sound inauthentic.
• Validate the client's experience and avoid prescribing your own solutions.
• Problems that appear complex might not require a complex solution.
• In wet weather we find dry wood within a log and focus on growing a fire from it, as we would listen for exceptions and instances of a preferred future already in existence. |

(Continued)

Table 4.2 Principles of Leave No Trace for Solution-Focused Outdoor Therapy (Cont'd)

Leave No Trace	Outdoor Practice	General Therapeutic Practice	Solution-Focused Practice
Respect Wildlife	• Do not chase, intimidate, or damage fauna and flora. • Keep disturbance, through noise for example, minimal.	• Respect everything our client brings to the session. • Do not take anything away from a session without clear permission.	• Recognize everything the client brings, especially ways to survive, their perseverance, and determination for a better future. • Tread lightly, conscientiously, and with respect.
Be Considerate to Other Visitors	• Be polite and considerate to other trail users, campsite users, river access and egress points. Give way to smaller or faster groups. Keep noise to a minimum at night.	• Be considerate to other stakeholders important to our clients.	• Respect others supplying third person narratives. • Be aware of solution-forced influences.

the impact practitioners have with those they work with. Most of us entered the field to contribute to such change. However, we remain mindful of respecting people's autonomy, dignity, knowledge, self-determination, and human rights. In emphasizing these aspects of human experience, the role of the practitioner decreases, while the role of the client amplifies. We do not go around planting our flags in our clients' lives.

Conclusion

Building on the tools for the solution-focused worker, this chapter presented how host leadership, experiential learning, and a novel ethical framework, grounded by sustainability ethics, can inform solution-focused practice outdoors. We argued this stance could inform clinically trained psychotherapists and those professionals working intentionally in outdoor environments. In the following chapter, we examine considerations for working with individual co-adventurers, considering the traditional one-hour session to the full day adventure. The following chapters take us into the weeds. We start the first session with individuals and take into consideration working with key stakeholders, such as parents and referrers.

References

Association for Experiential Education (2021). *About the AEE certified clinical adventure therapy credential (CCAT)*. Retrieved from www.aee.org/about-the-certification-program

Australian Association for Bush Adventure Therapy, Inc. [AABAT]. (2021). *About AABAT*. Retrieved from https://aabat.org.au/about-aabat/

Australian Association of Social Workers [AASW]. (2020). *Code of ethics*. www.aasw.asn.au/document/item/13400

Caldwell, B. E. (2015). *Saving psychotherapy: How therapists can bring the talking cure back from the brink*. Ben Caldwell Labs.

DeMille, S., Tucker, A. R., Gass, M. A., Javorski, S., VanKanegan, C., Talbot, B., & Karoff, M. (2018). The effectiveness of outdoor behavioral healthcare with struggling adolescents: A comparison group study a contribution for the special issue: Social innovation in child and youth services. *Children and Youth Services Review*, 88, 241–248. https://doi.org/10.1016/j.childyouth.2018.03.015

Dobud, W. W. (2020). *Experiences of adventure therapy: A narrative inquiry* [Doctoral Dissertation]. Charles Sturt University.

Dobud, W. W. (2021). Experiences of secure transport in outdoor behavioral healthcare: A narrative inquiry. *Qualitative Social Work*. https://doi.org/10.1177 %2F14733250211020088

Dobud, W. W., & Harper, N. J. (2018). Of dodo birds and common factors: A scoping review of direct comparison trials in adventure therapy. *Complementary Therapies in Clinical Practice, 31*, 16–24. https://doi.org/10.1016/j.ctcp.2018.01.005

Duncan, B. L. (2014). *On becoming a better therapist: Evidence-based practice one client at a time*. American Psychological Association.

Duncan, B. L., Hubble, M. A., & Miller, S. D. (2004). Beyond integration: The triumph of outcome over process in clinical practice. *Psychotherapy in Australia, 10*(2), 2–19.

Egan, G. (2002). *The skilled helper* (7th ed.) Brooks/Cole.

European Court of Human Rights. (1998). *European convention on human rights*. Council of Europe. Retrieved from www.echr.coe.int/documents/convention_eng.pdf

European Mentoring and Coaching Council. (2016). *Global code of ethics*. Retrieved from www.emccglobal.org/leadership-development/ethics/

Frank, J. D., & Frank, J. B. (1991). *Persuasion and healing: A comparative study of psychotherapy*. JHU Press.

Gelso, C. J., Kivlighan, D. M., Jr., & Markin, R. D. (2018). The real relationship and its role in psychotherapy outcome: A meta-analysis. *Psychotherapy, 55*(4), 434–444. https://doi.org/10.1037/pst0000183

Gray, D. E. (2011). Journeys towards the professionalisation of coaching: Dilemmas, dialogues and decisions along the global pathway. *Coaching: An International Journal of Theory, Research and Practice, 4*(1), 4–19. https://doi.org/10.1080/17 521882.2010.550896

Greenleaf, R. K. (1970). *The servant as leader*. Greenleaf Publishing Centre.

Howard, K. I., Kopta, S. M., Krause, M. S., & Orlinsky, D. E. (1986). The dose–effect relationship in psychotherapy. *American Psychologist, 41*(2), 159–164. https://doi.org/10.1037/0003-066X.41.2.159

Howard, K. I., Lueger, R. J., Maling, M. S., & Martinovich, Z. (1993). A phase model of psychotherapy outcome: Causal mediation of change. *Journal of Consulting and Clinical Psychology, 61*(4), 678–685. https://doi.org/10.1037/0022-006X.61.4.678

Howard, K. I., Moras, K., Brill, P. L., Martinovich, Z., & Lutz, W. (1996). Evaluation of psychotherapy: Efficacy, effectiveness, and patient progress. *American Psychologist, 51*(10), 1059–1064. https://doi.org/10.1037/0003-066X.51.10.1059

Karoff, M., Tucker, A. R., Alvarez, T., & Kovacs, P. (2017). Infusing a peer-to-peer support program with adventure therapy for adolescent students with autism spectrum disorder. *Journal of Experiential Education*, 40(4), 394–408.

Khele, S., Symons, C., & Wheeler, S. (2008). An analysis of complaints to the British Association for Counselling and Psychotherapy, 1996–2006. *Counselling and Psychotherapy Research*, 8(2), 124–132. https://doi.org/10.1080/14733140802051408

Loynes, C. (1998). Adventure in a bun. *Journal of Experiential Education*, 21(1), 35–39. https://doi.org/10.1177%2F105382599802100108

McKergow, M., & Bailey, H. (2014). *Host: Six new roles of engagement for teams, organisations, communities and movements*. Solution Books.

McKergow, M., & Pugliese, P. (Eds.) (2019). *The host leadership field book: Building engagement for performance and results*. Solution Books.

Miller, S. D., Hubble, M. A., Chow, D. L., & Seidel, J. A. (2013). The outcome of psychotherapy: Yesterday, today, and tomorrow. *Psychotherapy*, 50(1), 88–97. https://doi.org/10.1037/a0031097

Mitten, D. (1994). Ethical considerations in adventure therapy: A feminist critique. *Women & Therapy*, 15(3–4), 55–84. https://doi.org/10.1300/J015v15n03_06

Natynczuk, S. (2016). *Perceptions of professionalism in adventure therapy: Working towards a competency framework* [Masters Dissertation]. University of Worcester.

Natynczuk, S. (2019). Host leadership in outdoor, bush, wilderness and adventure therapy. In M. McKergow and P. Pugliese (Eds.), *The host leadership field book: Building engagement for performance and results* (pp. 42–52). Solution Books.

Natynczuk, S., & Dobud, W. W. (2021). Leave no trace, willful unknowing, and implications from the ethics of sustainability for solution-focused practice outdoors. *Journal of Solution Focused Practices*, 5(2), 7.

Norcross, J. C., & Lambert, M. J. (2011). Psychotherapy relationships that work II. *Psychotherapy*, 48(1), 4–8. https://doi.org/10.1037/a0022180

Perske, R. (1972). The dignity of risk and the mentally retarded. *Mental Retardation*, 10(1), 24–27.

Pringle, G., Dobud, W. W., & Harper, N. J. (2021). The next frontier: Wilderness therapy and the treatment of complex trauma. In E. Brymer, M. Rogerson, & J. Barton (Eds.), *Nature and health: Physical activity in nature* (pp. 191–207). Routledge.

Ritzer, G. (1996, 2001). *Explorations in social theory*. SAGE Publications.

Roberts, J. W. (2005). Disney, Dewey, and the death of experience in education. *Education and Culture*, 21(2), 12–30.

Rogers, C. R. (1957). The necessary and sufficient conditions of therapeutic personality change. *Journal of Consulting Psychology, 21*(2), 95–103. https://doi.org/10.1037/h0045357

Stevenson, R. L. (1881). *Virginibus Puerisque*. Chatto and Windus.

Substance Abuse and Mental Health Services Administration [SAMHSA]. (2021). *SAMHSA – Substance Abuse and Mental Health Services Administration*. Retrieved from www.samhsa.gov/

United Nations (1948). *Universal declaration of human rights*. Retrieved from www.un.org/en/universal-declaration-human-rights/

Walsh, V., & Golins, G. (1976). *The exploration of the Outward Bound process*. Colorado Outward Bound School.

Wampold, B. E., & Imel, Z. E. (2015). *The great psychotherapy debate: The evidence for what makes psychotherapy work* (2nd ed.). Routledge.

5
Working with Individual Clients

"It's less about getting the words just right and more about holding to the fundamental belief that you don't know what's going on with the other person."

Bradford and Robin (2021, p. 111)

You are wrapping up a busy day at work. On the way home, you get on your bike, in your car, or on the bus. You are feeling quite hungry. Maybe you call a friend or your partner and ask them if they would like to go out for a meal. They agree to meet you at the restaurant. You arrive and the maître d' greets you. When welcomed, you let the maître d' know you would like a table for two, despite not having made a reservation. The maître d' reaches below the stand and pulls out a clipboard with paper attached. First, you and your guests are asked to complete five pages of paperwork. Allergies, dietary requirements, previous medical emergencies; it is covering a lot of information, and upon returning the questionnaire you then receive a barrage of questions about what brings you to the restaurant. "How long have you been hungry? Can you describe your hunger? Is this hunger related to any adverse childhood experiences?" The maître d' thanks you for providing the information and ducks back to the kitchen to talk with the chef. Upon returning, you are escorted to a table without menus and informed that the kitchen staff will bring you your meal shortly, based on the information you provided about the problem: *your hunger*.

We have liked this metaphor since we first heard it from Bannink (2010) and there are many more metaphors about the potential for problem-focused approaches missing the point. How about a taxi driver who focuses on your need for a ride without asking where you want to go? You would probably not enter the cab, let alone get to your preferred destination.

Aspects of this practice could be adopted and used as adjuncts to already established models of practice. In this chapter, we present specific approaches

DOI: 10.4324/9781003217558-7

to adopting an outdoor solution-focus while working with individual clients. Many practitioners worldwide are already implementing experiential modalities to their practice. For example, Tucker and Norton (2013) surveyed a random sample of over 600 clinical social workers in the United States finding more than a third to report using some sort of adventure-based activities in their practice. Our close friends and colleagues Harper et al. (2019) wrote a comprehensive and fantastic text on their approach to working with young people and family in nature-based therapy settings. This section is simply a different orientation based on solution-focused assumptions.

We broke this chapter up to show how we go about organizing our sessions. We start with the initial meeting and then look to subsequent sessions. Finding consensus between us about what this looks like raised interesting debates. Stepping away from the solution-focused model for a second, we must acknowledge that each practitioner brings their own flavor to not only their first session, but the entire therapeutic interaction. For Miller et al. (2013), removing the contributions of the therapist from understanding what is happening in the therapy setting would do violence to the phenomena of psychotherapy. We pay close attention to context and how co-adventurers experience the work, over and above the techniques we use (Wampold & Imel, 2015).

In the sections that follow, we examine considerations for increasing engagement in the first session. We revisit host leadership and why we inquire about pretreatment changes. Examples from our practice are included to examine how we can be more responsive when working with individuals in the outdoors.

Initial Sessions

I (Stephan) will often meet a co-adventurer at their home or school. Ideally, I will have a pre-session meeting where we talk about what our days together could look like. Some schools have funded full day sessions for introductions, other agencies favor a one- to two-hour meeting before any adventuring begins. We complete consent forms and go through the things the client should and need not bring along; for example, bring spare clothes, medication, and food for the day. Parents or carers are preferably involved in the pre-session meeting, and we talk about our hopes for the work together. The first session could be called a walk and talk. No specialist equipment is taken except what would normally be in an instructor's rucksack: spare top, hat and gloves, food, facility to provide a hot drink, flint, steel and birch bark, emergency shelter or a tarp, a comprehensive first aid kit, sunscreen, short rope, sling and karabiner, head-torches, knife, whistle, fully charged phone, map and compass, and bag for rubbish. Visit the First Session Checklist included in our field manual (Appendix H).

Active engagement starts from the word "go." We head off to somewhere not too far away where there is a hill, some forest, perhaps a river. These settings are referred to as *near-by nature* as opposed to remote, outdoor settings sometimes described as wilderness (Harper et al., 2019). My favorite first session venue is a forest where there are simple caves – easy to walk into darkness and out without the need for crawling or anything other than a short scramble, clifftop views, the chance of seeing wildlife, such as bats, deer, and spiders, and the reassuring footprints of other human explorers. I have a route in mind that introduces aspects of all the adventure activities I am qualified and licensed to lead. During the session, I make assessments of the participant's abilities to move over rough ground, their propensity for adventure, and sense of responsible leadership – their *adventurosity*.

Sometimes such a day in the forest is the first time a student has been away from their local urban environment, a significantly novel experience and potentially challenging by itself. The initial conversation as we leave the car is about contracting. They will not be forced into any activity, any adventure we set out on is optional and, when safe to do so, can be ended at any time. The possibility of stopping and ending a session, whatever we are doing, is available whenever they choose. Confidentiality is agreed unless there is indication that harm will be done to themselves, others, or property, and the regulations for referring my concerns to senior management or beyond to other authorities are understood.

Most importantly, it seems, is our discussion about roles and responsibilities. We are equal during the adventure in terms of looking out for each other and keeping each other safe from harm. We are co-adventurers with mutual responsibilities. While I might have the technical knowledge and experience to keep us safe, accidents happen and it might be them, the co-adventurer, who must call for rescue or stay to help the casualty. There is a chance that it could be the practitioner who gets injured. Everyone has a voice in contributing to the dynamic risk assessment and is listened to seriously.

Choices about what we do are shared and acted on collectively. Remember the Crucial C's. These conversations establish mutual respect and responsibility, and emphasize the spirit of co-adventuring. This seems to be fundamental in constructing a new dynamic for many outdoor therapy participants. Their input and leadership will be not only expected, it is taken seriously.

Contracting is the first step in living a solution-focused process, not just the formal agreements and understanding about confidentiality, the agreement and understanding of what the client wants from the work together.

Many outdoor therapies draw heavily on experiential education making, in many ways, the therapy is experiential beyond the conversation (Natynczuk, 2021). Practitioners watch out for exceptions to the client's everyday challenges. Practitioners notice the difference small things can make. Adventurous journeys are an unspoken metaphor for change and growth. The idea that an adventure is an undertaking with an uncertain outcome is very helpful: the work, the experiences, and their outcome are uncertain. We explore together, through which the participant enjoys the chance to gain some mastery, have different stories to tell, draw on inner resources and strengths, and altogether increase their social capital.

Initial conversations focus on establishing a climate of confidence, exploring what the client is good at, and what they enjoy doing. Practitioners may ask, "What do you enjoy doing most, what makes you happy?" We talk about their skills, knowledge and what brings them joy. With adolescents, we may ask when they are at their best. A favorite of ours is: "Think about the photos in your phone, is there a picture you could describe that shows you at your best?"

This question was used with a young person who left home due to domestic violence at a young age. At 16 years old, she lived in her car in various parking lots near the beach. When she was asked this question, at 22 years old, she responded that pictures of her at the beach were illustrative of her best self. We moved our sessions to the beach environment and spent time snorkeling at the reef. She described feeling free and independent when near the water, as she did when she bravely left home. She obtained full-time employment and enjoyed the sunset every night from her apartment balcony on the esplanade. Information about when our co-adventurers are at their best provides clues for tailoring our services.

First sessions can take place indoors. For individual sessions, we might give participants pictures of various activities we can do together, from rock climbing to caving, hiking to snorkeling, or journeying by canoe. We also suggest the opportunity to remain inside if they prefer. It is important to remember that this is *their* adventure and not ours. Some clients may like their sessions to remain indoors, or a mix of both. For many adolescents who have experienced a therapist's couch without benefit, doing something different could light a fire beneath them so to speak. The important task is asking useful questions to explore the potential therapeutic value of the future experience.

Go with the answer. Solution-focused approaches distance themselves from other models of therapy based on our initial encounter. The first session is no time for assessment beyond physical abilities and psychological concerns of safety. It is the start of the intervention all together (Ratner et al., 2012). Practitioners have a myriad of techniques related to evoking change and co-constructing a client's preferred future in relation to a life in which the problem brought to therapy is no longer present: a different way of being. Examples included in this section are discussions about pretreatment changes, the use of the tomorrow question, or simply asking about the co-adventurer's best hopes. What follows, however, is how we view ourselves as *hosts* of people's therapy experiences.

Being a Good Host

While some clients, especially youth or those referred for substance misuse, are unlikely to voluntarily seek our services (Sparks et al., 2007), we maintain our therapeutic assumptions. There is no such thing as an unmotivated client, at least we have yet to meet one, and we take full responsibility in rolling with their engagement in the therapeutic process. It is unlikely that anyone would go to therapy because they want things to get worse. As mentioned in Chapter 3, resistance is *not* a useful concept in therapy (Selekman, 2005) and we need to focus on our role as host of each outdoor therapy encounter.

A fantastic and resource-filled book for problems in initial therapy sessions written by Dr. Daryl Chow (2018), an Australian clinical psychologist and important voice around improving psychotherapy outcomes, is *The First Kiss: Undoing the Intake Model and Igniting First Sessions in Psychotherapy*. In this easy-to-read text, Chow addresses many of the problems occurring in psychotherapy, specifically around first sessions. He presents the differences between an intake model and the engagement model. While we present below some of the strategies for incorporating solution-focused techniques to a first session, we build on Chow's work and explore considerations for igniting first sessions in outdoor therapy.

Chow (2018) argued for dismantling the *Intake Model* by fixating on "being a good host" (p. 13). Practitioners are encouraged to adopt an *Engagement Model* in which strategies are utilized to improve the quality of the therapeutic relationship and provide experiences of success and mastery. It has been an error in judgment to treat our initial interactions with people as a *taking* instead of a *giving*. For many, first therapy sessions involve disclosing personal information to a stranger vacant of any focus on how this therapy helps. The practitioner (in)takes, the participant gives. We aim to turn this around. Where many practitioners are trained to screen or assess a client, we assess the first session based on engagement and our plans to work together. Instead of focusing on the problem bringing a client to therapy, we listen for their preferences. If we do not, we run the risk of getting stuck.

Baldwin et al. (2009) and Hansen et al. (2002) found the most common number of sessions people attend is *one*. This, of course, requires unpacking. Some brief therapists may believe the client received what they needed from one session and decided there was no need to return. Being an optimistic view for sure, the evidence found in the aforementioned studies suggested those who benefitted from the initial session were actually more likely to return for future sessions. For Chow (2018), practitioners should worry less about *their* intake and more about the client's experience in our care. Clients should leave the first session with hope they are already heading in the right direction.

There is a funny paradox to working with many of the adolescents referred to outdoor therapy services. They are sent for substance abusing, self-harming, disengaging from school, opposition, and a myriad of problematic behaviors. Parents may ask for a "wake up call" or another idiom which expects the therapist to place visible boundaries around the child's risk-taking behaviors. If this has not worked in the school setting or home, it is unlikely to work in the therapy setting. More of the same is likely to be followed by the same demoralization that brought them to therapy in the first place. The first session and interaction must be experienced positively by a client. We ask for feedback, not only to help ourselves get better at what we do. We want to model that we are interested in being useful, no matter what it looks like. We recommend checking in with a client halfway through the first session. If they have seen previous therapists, ask them how this session compares, are they getting what they need? Therapists should not be looking for plaudits for their impact. Transparency and an openness to feedback are key.

I (Will) consulted with an alternative school in a rural and remote Australian town. I was referred a 16-year-old student named, for this account, as Rosie who was a survivor of horrific, violent trauma, self-harmed on a regular basis, and lived with disengaged parents. As we sat in the government-funded school, with couches way too low to the ground, I remember thinking how uncomfortable and awkward this session was. And I was not the client! "I've done this before," she would say. "Everyone thinks I just need to talk. I don't want to talk." I filmed this session, and at about the 45-minute mark, Rosie said she was learning to play the drums from a friend of hers. In the video, you can see my back straighten as I lean towards her with excitement. After talking about how good of a resource her friend sounded, I shared that I had been playing the drums since I was five years old. We immediately bounced to our feet and ran to the music room. From then on, our sessions took place in the music room. We mastered inspirational punk rock songs of her choosing. Rosie on drums, I on guitar and vocals. Rosie started talking about not wanting to self-harm anymore. The school principal noticed Rosie arrived on time and engaged with her studies. She was also becoming a leader on LGBTQ+ issues and spoke to students about the effects of sexual assault and discrimination. Like many of these roles, management changed and the principal who hired me for consultation left taking me with her to another agency in need of a new voice and perspective. Rosie sent the principal a Christmas card thanking her for putting us in touch with each other. While not outdoors, I like to use this certainly experiential case example as an opportunity for following our co-adventurers' lead, especially when I felt lost for the first 45 minutes of the session.

No matter how prepared we are for a session, whether the first or twentieth, ruptures occur. Repairing ruptures is important, requiring skill and humility. We discuss some of this work further along in this chapter. In the following sections, we will begin to unpack the areas of focus used in our outdoor solution-focused practice.

Structuring the First Session

There are many ways to conduct a first session. We will link to some of the classic solution-focused techniques with our outdoor work to describe the potential of pretreatment changes, using the tomorrow question, and finding exceptions to uncover clues for unique outcomes and the client's best hopes. These techniques can also be used in groups and expedition settings, as well as with parents or referring parties.

Pretreatment Changes

Freud (2012) found many of the people he was seeing to experience what he referred to as a "flight to health" early on in therapy and even prior to their first session. He hypothesized this sudden change was due to a pathological failure to deal with the problems bringing the person to therapy. For the solution-focused practitioner, pretreatment changes occur when the first session is booked. Ratner et al. (2012) suggested that the:

> obvious answer is not that the client has taken a flight to health but rather, on committing himself to the possibility of a solution, finds himself, perhaps unconsciously, open to new and different thoughts about the problem and is thus more likely to find a solution.
>
> (p. 58)

We do present, in Chapter 7, our process for working with families and other referrers, and these questions can be perfect for them. For example, practitioners can thank a parent or school counselor for the referral and ask them to take note of any changes occurring between then and the next appointment. They might ask for signs of hope that things are heading in the right direction. Simply put, practitioners explore what changes people notice between the time of booking the first session and when they arrive for it. Weiner-Davis et al. (1987) found roughly 70% of clients were able to describe some pretreatment changes during their initial session.

Outdoor solution-focused practitioners draw on pretreatment changes in their work. If a co-adventurer reports standing up to a problem, or feeling happier, we ask how they were able to do it or what they noticed about themselves at that time. Their response helps consolidate gains and build meaning around their capabilities and resources. We can then ask what we will notice if they continue enacting change this way during the experiential outdoor session. For example, if a co-adventurer describes how their body posture changed when they were able to stand up to distressing thoughts, we might ask how they can practice that throughout the walk and talk session in the forest. Pretreatment changes are clues practitioners build on. The questions we ask and activities we facilitate build on the strengths and changes co-adventurers have already enacted in their lives.

The Miracle or Tomorrow Question and the Client's Best Hopes

The miracle or, for those not happy with miracles, the tomorrow question is arguably the most popular solution-focused intervention. It was formulated by Insoo Kim Berg as she sat with a client struggling to imagine a hopeful future. The client told Insoo that "maybe only a miracle will help." Along with de Shazer (1988), the two recognized that asking clients about a miraculous change can help with lifting them out of self-defeating notions that no change is possible. Historically, the question has been framed something like this:

> I'm going to ask you a rather strange question [pause]. The strange question is this: [pause] After we talk, you will go back to your work (home, school) and you will do whatever you need to do the rest of today, such as taking care of children, cooking dinner, watching TV, giving the children a bath, and so on. It will be time to go to bed. Everybody in your household is quiet, and you are sleeping in peace. In the middle of the night, a miracle happens and the problem that prompted you to talk to me today is solved! But because it happens while you are sleeping, you have no way of knowing that there was an overnight miracle that solved the problem [pause]. So, when you wake up tomorrow morning, what might be the small change that will make you say to yourself, "Wow, something must have happened – the problem is gone!"?
>
> (Berg & Dolan, 2001, p. 7)

Each practitioner brings their own style to the miracle question based on their clientele and the client's presentation. The miracle question and other solution-focused techniques have evolved due to the work of other practitioners and advocates. Questions similar to the miracle question emerged. For example, George et al. (1990) started their initial sessions asking, "So, what are your best hopes from our talking together" (p. 13). The purpose of this question, as put by Natynczuk (2014), is to "establish what the client wants to achieve for himself and… his best hopes for the conversation" (p. 27). We ask our clients each encounter about their best hopes for the day. In outdoor therapy, we might hear something about an activity we have been doing, such as a climb, a cave, or a river trip. Sometimes it is to talk. Occasionally, it is to pursue a personal development gain. One co-adventurer I (Stephan) recently took on his first overnight mountain climb asked if this trip would make him more resilient. Naturally, I was delighted by this question, which became the topic of conversation as we climbed to the summit. We explored all the signs of increased resilience we would notice during and after the trip, and what difference they would make.

If we look back to the theoretical positions of this approach, you will notice a philosophical shift in how we view the people coming to us for help. To avoid being repetitive, we are not going to discuss that further, but instead discuss some of the concerns we have heard from practitioners who have attended our workshops. The first one being, if the client is externally motivated to therapy by their family, school, or the court system, how can they know their best hopes? Second, what if their response to the miracle question is unrealistic? Third, what if someone does not know what they want?

Working with "Involuntary" Clients

While adventure therapy, and wilderness therapy in the United States in particular (Tucker et al., 2015, 2018), has aspects of involuntary and coercive practice that we do not condone as per our own professional ethics, we do wish to reflect on the nature of involuntary treatment. Imagine the mother or father of a 15-year-old growing concerned as their child was caught with marijuana at school. The school has threatened to expel the young man if he does not seek therapy services from you. A week later, the boy gets in the car with his parents, drives to wherever it is you work, maybe sits in a waiting room, completes necessary paperwork, and under his own power, enters your office. Of course, coercion is possible in this example. What differentiates our view of a mandated client is that there is always a motivation to improve someone's situation. It is likely that if someone turns up, they want something. It is unlikely someone arriving to therapy is actively trying to make things worse. This young person's best hopes could simply be not being thrown out of school or getting his parents off his back. In this case, we will know the session may be useful if the client is able to remain in school and if his parents are off his back.

Those who have worked with "involuntary" young people may be used to clients saying they do not have best hopes for a session since they are just attending because someone forced them to. The difference is we do not see therapy as a treatment to fix a disorder, which is something done to someone in the expectation of curing them. We do not agree with therapy including punitive elements with the aim of coercion or compliance. Clients are welcomed as proactive in finding their own solutions to whatever brought them into therapy. The case example below looks at how we can work to greet someone disinterested in coming to therapy.

Charlie's wife was unhappy he was caught drunk driving. He drove for a living and lost his job. Knowing that Charlie loved fishing with his friends from work, his wife found a psychologist in their community who worked outdoors. She told Charlie to go and meet the practitioner at his office to make a plan. At the first session, Charlie's best hopes were to make his wife happy. He was adamant he was not an alcoholic and just made this one mistake. Resisting the urge to simply ask more questions about his drinking, the psychologist asked when Charlie was at his best. He described his love of fly fishing. "What do you notice about yourself when you're fishing that makes a difference?" the psychologist asked. Charlie described feeling peace and moments of restoration. The two agreed those moments are important and arranged to meet at a winding river trail for their next session.

After a few sessions, Charlie invited his wife to the next session and said he hoped they could spend more time together outdoors, instead of heavily drinking each weekend.

Many are coerced to therapy, and even more may arrive with little faith in its effectiveness. An exception to the problem that brought Charlie to therapy was his love of being outside. His best hopes related to improving his relationship with his wife, which might address his drinking, though was not the terminology or preference he had for making things better. The psychologist inquired about what difference being outside meant to Charlie, rather than focusing on the problem. Inquiring into the problematic drinking would have fulfilled Charlie's belief that the psychologist was simply an extension of his wife, working towards her best hopes, leaving Charlie invalidated, and the problem alive. Moving on from the problem, looking for signs of change rather than generating a set of tasks means we are moving towards a satisfactory solution.

The option of taking therapy outdoors can make our co-adventurers feel less threatened by the obvious and inherent power differential that comes with therapy. We sit side by side, walk shoulder to shoulder, or even sit behind each other in a canoe. Maintaining our solution-focused assumptions, specifically about motivation, requires discipline. We do not view ourselves as psychotherapists on a white stallion parading into someone's life as experts in their lived experiences or best hopes, with all the answers we think our client needs. Doing so invites disengagement as the client must defend their worldview. Someone's best hopes and resources may look nothing like the preferred future of the referrer. They are indicators practitioners use to focus their work and improve engagement. As our alliance strengthens, we may be able to talk about the impact of someone's drinking, if necessary, and if the client asks. Stick with building a climate of competence and allow the outdoor session to be the very exception to the problem people can build on in the future.

Can Someone's Best Hopes Be Unrealistic?

If we are true to the concept of working in our client's best interests, we must take them at their word and trust them as experts on themselves. We avoid judgments of what is realistic or not for them in the same way that we would not presume to know what is positive or beneficial. Good use of solution-focused tools prompts co-adventurers to add realism to their best hopes. As Bradford and Robin (2021) described at the start of this chapter, practitioners are encouraged to focus less on specific techniques, lengthy bio-psychosocial assessments, or asking the right question at the right time, and more on the client's best hopes, motivation, and preferences while appreciating that we are not experts in their lived experience.

Sometimes best hopes are too far in the future. Our work should bring the client to a point in the near future when it is more likely that the differences small changes make can be made real. Those small changes come from our use of scales, questions of difference, explorations of exceptions, others' perceptions of change, and our use of "suppose" in the tomorrow or miracle question.

While sitting with a 21-year-old in an anchored canoe in the beautiful mangroves of Garden Island in South Australia, I (Will) was caught off guard by an interesting statement. "None of this would have ever happened if my mother was still alive," he said as he cast his fishing line back into the water. He was referred to me for a destructive relationship with his father and increasing substance use. We had already worked together for a few indoor counseling sessions, but this was the first time we were outdoors. Of course, I could not bring his mother back. He had never mentioned his mother before. I acknowledged his pain and attempted to validate how difficult things must have been. I then asked, "What difference would it make if your mother was around?"

"I wouldn't be doing any of this shit, the drugs, the fighting," he responded. We talked about what difference it would make if he was not doing these things and what those around him would notice, starting with his father and siblings. "We would be a happy family again. We would have dinner together around the table and talk about our day like we used to with mom."

Our next session, he reported to have made dinner for the family on three occasions. His father reported improved communication and less fighting. Despite the client's very best hopes being "unrealistic," the differences they could have made led to a unique outcome driven from a line of solution-focused questioning.

Do People Really Know What They Want?

It is a fair assumption, and a solution-focused assumption, that people generally want something to be better and there are only a miniscule number who deliberately want things to be worse. Guy Shennan (2019) talks about two simple assumptions we can make: 1) if someone is seeking help then there must be something wrong; and 2) if someone has gone to another person for help, then they must have hope for something useful to come from this effort. Shennan described the first as a problem-focused assumption, the second a solution-focused assumption. If someone wants something to be better our role as solution-focused practitioners is to ask what it is they want. Trust co-adventurers to know what they want and travel therapeutically together in the most useful direction possible. Our collective aim is in describing and experiencing desired outcomes and eliciting descriptions of what a preferred destination will look like when we arrive. The description of this "place" is entirely the clients'. It is not for the practitioner to decide. A metaphor for this is catching a bus that does not go to exactly the place we want to be, close enough the difference matters little.

Taking the Therapy Outside: Looking for Possibilities and Stretching the World

McKergow's (2021) book on the next generation of solution-focused practice talks about stretching a client's world rather than changing or rebuilding it. Putting this idea into an outdoor context is interesting: a stretch requires effort from a co-adventurer, new thinking takes time and effort, and new experiences have to be weighed and reflected upon. The stretch might mean returning to the original world size. We cannot say how long the stretch will last, though with a world already stretched from our work together, there is space for something different in between the old and the new. At the next session, the follow up question of "What's better?" is a way of asking how the newly stretched world is working.

Iain is happy for us to use his real name. He was referred to me (Stephan) because of other practitioners' concerns around his travel anxieties being a block to attending school. I went to visit Iain in the small market town where he was living independently to talk about what we could do that might be helpful. We seemed to get along well in our initial conversations. "So, what adventure would you like to do during our time together?" I asked.

"Caving" replied Iain. His enthusiasm was certainly tangible.

"Fantastic," I replied genuinely. There were no caves or mines we could explore within an hour's drive of where he lived. We never actually spoke about travel or any challenges that might come about because of it. We simply went caving each week for the summer with a few days camping on several occasions so we could travel further afield and explore more demanding cave systems. The problem was never spoken about and the solution, traveling for a purpose we enjoyed, was lived. One might argue the stretch persisted. After the summer Iain attended college. The journey was not straightforward. A lift was required from a parent, then a train had to be caught, and a bus trip for the last section. At the end of the day the three-part journey was repeated in reverse. Iain attended college and then took his work experience in my private practice, eventually becoming a trainee and an employee. Iain now works as an underground adventure guide.

Subsequent Sessions

In classic solution-focused practice, every session, including the first, could be the last. Every subsequent one is a follow-up where we examine the changes that occurred between sessions. For many, this is the week-to-week therapy they grow accustomed to, though we aim only for as many sessions as the client prefers and not one more (Ratner et al., 2012).

Some practitioners may begin a subsequent session asking clients how their week has gone. A solution-focused practitioner is more direct and asks, "What is better since we last met?" At this stage in a workshop or training, we start to see therapists' hands getting raised. "Isn't this an assumption?" one may ask. "What if things aren't better?"

Solution-focused therapy is rooted in social construction and therapists and clients co-construct change together through their conversations. This is not to undermine the tight rope we walk attending to a person's wounded humanity while gently pointing to progressive narratives. Asking a client what is better since the last meeting invites a "progressive" or solution-focused narrative. de Shazer (1991), for example, theorized that "solution-determined (progressive) narratives are more likely than complaint-centered narratives… to produce transformations and discontinuities" (p. 92). The question is designed to direct a client's attention. After a few weeks, co-adventurers start arriving to sessions saying, "I knew you were going to ask me that!" Put concisely by Ratner et al. (2012), "Watching out for what has been better is very specifically at the heart of the solution focused change process" (p. 149).

This question typically invites three responses: things got better, or worse, or nothing changed. The following sections will unpack these three possibilities. As we present in Chapter 9 about outcome monitoring, it is important to keep our relationship open to hearing about a lack of progress so we can adjust the therapy, never the person. Still, we direct our co-adventurers to contract a solution-determined narrative.

It is possible a mandated co-adventurer has done something wrong making them easy to judge. Practitioners are encouraged to seek clinical supervision if these thoughts and feelings arise. They are likely to impact a practitioners' genuineness, which can create a rupture to the therapeutic alliance. Due to previous therapeutic experiences, they may distrust the system, or therapy in general. Validate those concerns and maybe communicate a healthy skepticism of the system as well. If someone has experienced "bad therapy," it is not necessarily because they saw a bad therapist, but their experience held little meaning and there were issues in the alliance. Discussing previous experiences of therapy, practitioners acknowledge they hate when these things happen because it creates a negative stigma to our work, while also stressing this is why they are only interested in being useful and not working on anything but the client's preferred future.

Things Are Better

Every change, even the very smallest of changes, is helpful. It is important to respect the smallest particles of change as they demonstrate movement in the desired direction, and the potential for more. Minimizing the smallest of steps by trivializing their meaning reduces the likelihood of subsequent change. Even the biggest journey begins with the smallest of steps. Ratner et al. (2012) described two types of questions when it comes to clients talking about examples of their active agency: strategy questions and identity questions.

"How did you get yourself to do that?" is perhaps the most straightforward question we could ask when a client tells us of an instance of their preferred future. We check if they were pleased to be able to do it. We help by asking for the client to offer ten or more things they noticed about themselves on that occasion. An answer of "I just felt better" is an invitation for more respectful curiosity. "So, what have you noticed that leads to feeling better?" These are Ratner et al.'s (2012) strategic questions. They take a broad view and invite evidence for the direction someone is moving. We strengthen that evidence by inviting third person perspectives: "Who would notice these changes?" Followed by "and what would they have seen telling them things were getting better for you?"

When people report signs of improvement, we bring these actions to life experientially during the outdoor therapy session. As details are elicited about how the client made this happen, we search for signs of what we, the practitioner, would notice if the co-adventurer lived these successes during the session. For example, if a client reports resisting the urge to self-harm by stopping for a moment to engage in deep breathing, we ask how deep breathing could help during the caving or canoeing adventure they scheduled. Throughout the session, the practitioner amplifies this gain, a key exception to the problem, in order to strengthen the change.

Identity questions help clients make sense of themselves and construct a more manageable world. We listen for examples of achievements aligned to the client's best hopes for our work together, and ask them to notice and name qualities, strengths, skills, and competencies that support their competent self. Perhaps they will notice a stronger self, more capable than they realized. We can be curious about this too. "What difference will it make to your future now that you know you can be this strong?" Or "Tell me about times when you have been this strong before?"

No Change

When asked what has improved since our last meeting, it is possible clients respond with a frank "nothing" (Bannink, 2010). The question invites the participant to consider what is, in fact, better. Of course, maybe nothing has improved, though one can always find an exception when a problem is minimized or absent. Careful questioning and use of language is important here. It is not *whether* there were exceptions, it is *when*.

Practitioners may ask what the person did to ensure things did not get worse. These types of questions have been referred to as *pessimistic* questions (Selekman, 2005). The practitioner may ask, "How did you manage to maintain the current situation?" Ideally, a similar line of questioning can elicit coping strategies and resources you can draw on experientially during the outdoor therapy session.

Ben, 14 years old, was asked, "What's better?" during his second session of outdoor therapy. He indicated no change. He was still getting bullied at school. Funded by Ben's school, the practitioner organized a short walk into the woods to practice some campcraft. In their first session, Ben communicated interest in learning survival strategies, such as sparking a fire with a flint and steel. When asked about how he managed to prevent things from getting worse, Ben replied he was able to remain calm and collected, trying not to get frustrated or lash out. The practitioner continued inquiring about what difference this made as they walked to their bushcraft location.

It rained the night before and the practitioner knew Ben could struggle sparking the fire. He said,

> "It sounds like remaining calm and collected was important to making sure things didn't get worse this week. I know we're working on fire lighting today, which is really cool. It rained last night and sometimes people can get really frustrated learning to do this. I can give you some tips if you like. Often a log wet on the outside is dry on the inside. We can make kindling from there. It sounds like you are a calm and collected guy who can roll with the punches if it gets hard. What would I notice indicating you are being calm and collected?"

The practitioner aimed to bring any exception to the problem or resource into the co-adventurer's attention. We are inviting them to notice their strengths and apply them experientially to our outdoor therapy work. Creating a climate of competence where participants lean on their capabilities and coping strategies helps to magnify them. To close the session, practitioners can ask what worked for the co-adventurers and what difference it will make using these strategies in the future.

Things Are Worse

Some may tell us things are getting worse. They communicate this on outcome measures, in response to our scaling questions, or simply walk in, slump to the ground, and start describing the areas of their wellbeing in decline. If practitioners move too fast, clients might feel invalidated. If they move into an outdoor activity before allowing the space for open discussion, even when negative, a rupture to the alliance is indicated.

Practitioners should avoid becoming too optimistic when they hear things are getting worse (Bannink, 2010). Like scenarios where no change is indicated, it can be helpful to ask questions to externalize the problem or invite a colleague to consult with the practitioner and client about what changes can be made to the course of therapy.

"This is bullshit," Rachel declared. "I came here because people said it would help. Rachel had been seeing a youth worker for six sessions and when he asked what had been improving, Rachel finally voiced her frustration. Living in a youth residential care setting after being taken away from her parents due to early childhood neglect, Rachel was tired of adults over-promising miracle results. She found herself in trouble every night in the group home for severe self-harming and experienced no relief from the near 25 helping professions she was sent to. The workers in her facility removed the door from her bedroom and she was not allowed to shave or access to the kitchen. Any attempt to adopt a future focus, such as using the miracle question, felt like an insult. "Things aren't getting better," the worker said, attempting to validate Rachel's rightful concern. "I know there have been a lot of empty promises that this stuff will help you. I wonder if I can ask you what may be a weird question, because I do not want to make this mistake again. I believe you have so much experience and us therapy folks have a lot to learn from you to improve our field! If you were to deliver a training, what advice would you give professionals in a similar position to me? Don't hold back!"

"Stop just asking questions. Talking doesn't do anything when I live in this shithole! All these strategies people give me don't do shit. The workers are horrible to me, and I just can't live here anymore!" she explained. The worker inquired about what Rachel would notice if things changed. "I'd feel myself. That I can be myself."

After the session, the practitioner called the residential setting's manager and described what was going on. The practitioners arranged to join a case meeting next week to invite some of the workers on a hike with Rachel. They wanted to give the team a chance to see Rachel at her best, to change the way Rachel is treated and perceived. The practitioner explained this to Rachel, and she hesitantly agreed. Three of the staff members attended and Rachel demonstrated how she learned to choose the trails she wanted to hike and navigate with a map and compass.

Rachel's self-harming behavior put the workers on edge. They walked into the group home every day scared they would be the one on call when she took things too far. They communicated this to Rachel. "You don't treat me like I'm a human," Rachel responded with tears welling up. "It's bullshit. Everyone says they want to help but it's only to help themselves." The team apologized and the three residential care workers, the youth worker, Rachel, and the program director sat on top of the mountain agreeing to be more open with their communication. Rachel found doing something real together made her feel like she could approach these three workers if she were to feel the urge to self-harm in the future.

Practitioners are encouraged to ask, "What's better?" each subsequent session. While the question aims to direct a co-adventurer's attention to signs of change, it is important to respect the real possibility things are worse. Assuming a weekly therapy encounter is enough to facilitate widespread change is overly optimistic and practitioners should avoid becoming defensive when clients report a lack of progress or deterioration. The youth worker in this case took Rachel's concerns seriously and adjusted the therapy, stepping into the role of advocate to help privilege her best hopes of being "treated like a person." Adjust the therapy, not the person. When things are going badly for a co-adventurer we might tactfully enquire how they are coping. This turns a problem focus to a solution focus by bringing in strengths and helpful qualities.

Closing the Session

As solution-focused practice developed from the early days of Steve de Shazer and Berg (1997), there were many ideas about how we should conclude our sessions. Some years ago, the practitioner took a break from the 60-minute session, met with a team that observed the session behind a one-way mirror, and devised a clever homework intervention for the client to utilize when they left the session. Not only was the two-way mirror "rather creepy" (McKergow, 2016, p. 12), practitioners rarely work in teams now and there has been a shift in how practitioners wrap up their sessions with a future focus, avoiding the need to prescribe a list of tasks to the client as homework. This includes: 1) appreciative summarizing; 2) exploring the client's confidence; 3) eliciting feedback; and 4) discussing what to do about subsequent sessions.

Appreciative Summarizing

First, we focus on more *appreciative summarizing* (McKergow, 2016). Doing so communicates empathy to the client by offering the chance to demonstrate that, yes, we have been listening and listening well. We are also afforded some small creative license in which narrative we choose to reflect. Anything that helps the client to hone in on when even the smallest changes have occurred is useful. If during a caving session, your co-adventurer points out the feeling of peace and calm of sitting in the total quiet, you may ask if there are similar moments she has experienced in the past. She is not sure. You ask what she would notice if she started feeling this way at home. She begins describing a slowing heart rate, control of her breathing, and more space to think. When summarizing the session, you may describe this sense of calm, and how she may look out for signs for when she notices this feeling during the week. Since she experienced this feeling during the session, rich material exists for her to focus on during the week.

Shennan (2019) suggested summarizing with the client's own words, experiences, strengths, and exceptions, in preference to complimenting. Compliments risk the practitioner making judgments which compromise one's non-judgmental, unconditional position. With the removal of homework from solution-focused practice, task-focused compliments lose much of their role. Instead, we acknowledge difficulty, summarize qualities, strengths, and capacities clients bring to bear on the change they want, acknowledge action and movement in a desired direction, and summarize signs of hope. Most importantly, we want to identify the signs of experienced success, mastery, and a climate of confidence.

Confidence

During the session, practitioners explore participants' best hopes and preferred future in detail. They add to this any exceptions or moments of success and mastery they noticed during the session, such as that feeling of calm during the caving session or being able to work patiently while starting a fire in the rain. George (2017) described three ways practitioners can explore someone's confidence at the end of a session. After providing an appreciative summary, practitioners can explore the co-adventurer's confidence using the tools described below:

- Using a scale from 1–10, ask how confident co-adventurers are about making progress towards their best hopes. Examine why they feel so confident and what is fueling this level of confidence.
- If the co-adventurer reports positive changes between your adventures together, inquire about their confidence in maintaining this level of change, or the chance of further improvements. You can use a similar scale for this as well. If you are reaching the end of your work together, or closing an expedition, these questions may be useful for helping someone focus on their confidence of change as they return home.
- Ask about their confidence in relation to maintaining change. Despite having asked about their best hopes and preferred future, ask how they will know when they have reached a level that is *good enough*. This can help you to gauge progress.

Natalie is a 17-year-old referred by her parents for concerns relating to her eating habits and self-harming behaviors. You have organized a hike for your first session. As the trek begins, you ask about previous therapy experiences. She unloaded a barrage of horrifying, borderline unethical stories. You ask for best hopes for this therapy, of which there are little. Her confidence in your service is uncharacteristically low. However, Natalie touches on her climate anxiety and explains her concerns for the planet. She mentions attending a student climate protest the week before. You sense a climate of competence (pun intended) and intentionally ask more questions about her passion for saving the planet. As the two of you return to your starting point, Natalie declares, "You know, this was really fun. It is so different from anything I have done before!" You ask what others will notice if she was acting similarly at home. She tells you she would voice her concerns with the adults around her in a more receptive way. Her parents would worry less, the leading cause of conflict. To explore Natalie's confidence, you might ask: "If you communicated your passions this way, those around you may be more receptive to your concerns. On a scale from 0 to 10, how confident are you that you can make progress towards this?" Natalie replies with a 6. She never felt that therapy could work before, and never felt this way with a helping professional. You can now unpack what she notices that has allowed her to score a 6 and work with the scaling tool.

Eliciting Feedback

While we begin our sessions with a solution-focus, the feedback we elicit from our clients helps to tailor our approach to each person's unique preferences. Positive feedback is fine, and it is a good idea to keep a folder of the good feedback you acquire for your own self-care. However, negative feedback is best. It helps to improve our performance. If we are not improving and feeling like we are getting better, we are destined for burnout, similar to how we might cancel our gym membership when we plateau in our results.

We like to save five or ten minutes at the end of each session to elicit client feedback. If you are driving with a participant, the car ride after a day's adventure is the perfect time for these discussions. We like to ask co-adventurers what seemed particularly beneficial and what could have made our time together more meaningful. We inquire about what was missing. Giving negative feedback is hard. Asking for it even harder. We recommend working with a supervisor or coach to explore strategies for asking useful questions that help us get better at tailoring our practice to client feedback (Miller et al., 2020).

Planning Subsequent Sessions

Bannink (2010) used an example of the family doctor in comparing how solution-focused practitioners view their work. The doctor may schedule a visit after a patient has undergone a series of tests, or to ensure that the person is responding to the new prescribed medication. The doctor aims to help the patient yet knows she cannot prescribe a bill of perfect health. That is typically a lofty outcome going well beyond the patient's chief concern, such as relieving chest pain. Selekman (1993) informed this view, writing:

> I do not believe my job is to cure people, but instead, to help clients have more satisfactory life situations. If clients call to cancel future scheduled appointments because they feel things are better for the time being, I always let them know that I have an open door policy and if they need to schedule a future tune-up session, they may feel free to call me.
>
> (p. 156)

We avoid telling co-adventurers when to return for ongoing therapy. It is better if they schedule subsequent sessions themselves. While closing, we ask when would be useful, especially if our caseload is increasing and vacancies the following week are limited. We do not mind if people schedule as needed, which many adolescents seem to prefer once a strong alliance is established. In fact, we have had clients and parents reach out years later when troubles in their life seem worthy of further counseling.

Ask about the next session. Do not prescribe it. Notwithstanding people's time, some may open their wallets to see you. Never waste clients' time or money. Strive to be as efficient as possible and abstain from assuming that amounts of time that worked for one person will work for the next. For example, Gass et al. (2019) claimed the average length of stay at US wilderness therapy programs was 90 days. Change, however, typically occurs in therapy sooner rather than later (Miller et al., 2020). The decisions on how long to keep someone in care are seldom made on evidence from outcome or alliance measures. More effective therapy is good. The opposite rings true as well. When therapy is not working, more of the same is counterproductive.

Conclusion

Taking individual therapy outdoors is full of possibilities. Adopting a solution-focus invites practitioners to consider how they host experiences which facilitate client change. Co-adventurers may experience moments during a session that are exceptions to the very problem that brought them to therapy. Reflecting on the questions practitioners ask, they may leave the session attempting to notice the signs that indicate change is happening.

Though seemingly counterintuitive, solution-focused practitioners never work harder than their clients. This may not be the case when it comes to monitoring safety or facilitating a session on, for example, a busy crag, though practitioners should not want to reach a preferred future more than their client does. If we find ourselves in this situation, we are encouraged to revisit the person's best hopes and lean back to ask more open-ended questions (Bannink, 2010; Ratner et al., 2012). For Harper et al. (2019), one of the many affordances of outdoor therapies is practitioners having the chance to benefit from the restorative power of being in nature day in and day out. If co-adventurers go home with the energy to engage with their families and have fun, we should too! It is best when both the co-adventurer and the practitioner have energy after their session.

What differentiates the solution-focused approach we described here from other outdoor therapy pursuits is the focus on hosting a moment where people experience themselves at their best, while using empirically supported strategies to encourage reflection and a future focus. This work looks similar in group settings or while on an expedition, where hosting may take on even more importance. The following chapter examines considerations for these contexts.

References

Baldwin, S. A., Berkeljon, A., Atkins, D. C., Olsen, J. A., & Nielsen, S. L. (2009). Rates of change in naturalistic psychotherapy: Contrasting dose-effect and good-enough level models of change. *Journal of Consulting and Clinical Psychology*, 77(2), 203–211. https://doi.org/10.1037/a0015235

Bannink, F. (2010). *1001 solution-focused questions: Handbook for solution-focused interviewing*. W. W. Norton & Co.

Berg, I. K., & Dolan, Y. (2001). *Tales of solutions: A collection of hope-inspiring stories*. W. W. Norton & Co.

Bradford, D., & Robin, D. (2021). *Connect: Building exceptional relationships with family, friends, and colleagues*. Penguin UK.

Chow, D. (2018). *The first kiss: Undoing the intake model and igniting first sessions in psychotherapy*. Correlate Press.

de Shazer, S. (1988). *Clues: Investigating solutions in brief therapy*. W. W. Norton & Co.

de Shazer, S. (1991). *Putting difference to work*. W. W. Norton & Co.

de Shazer, S., & Berg, I. K. (1997). What works? Remarks on research aspects of solution-focused brief therapy. *Journal of Family Therapy, 19*(2), 121–124. https://doi.org/10.1111/1467-6427.00043

Freud, S. (2012). *The basic writings of Sigmund Freud*. Modern Library.

Gass, M., Wilson, T., Talbot, B., Tucker, A., Ugianskis, M., & Brennan, N. (2019). The value of outdoor behavioral healthcare for adolescent substance users with comorbid conditions. *Substance Abuse: Research and Treatment, 13*. https://doi.org/10.1177/1178221819870768

George, E. (2017). *Scaling up our practice*. BRIEF. Retrieved from www.brief.org.uk/blog/2017/05/04/scaling-up-our-practice/

George, E., Iveson, C., & Ratner, H. (1990). *Problem to solution: Brief therapy with individuals and families*. BT Press.

Hansen, N. B., Lambert, M. J., & Forman, E. M. (2002). The psychotherapy dose-response effect and its implications for treatment delivery services. *Clinical Psychology: Science and Practice, 9*(3), 329–343. https://doi.org/10.1093/clipsy.9.3.329

Harper, N. J., Rose, K., & Segal, D. (2019). *Nature-based therapy: A practitioner's guide to working outdoors with children, youth, and families*. New Society Publishers.

McKergow, M. (2016). SFBT 2.0: The next generation of solution-focused brief therapy has already arrived. *Journal of Solution-Focused Brief Therapy, 2*(2), 1–17.

McKergow, M. (2021). *The next generation of solution focused practice: Stretching the world for new opportunities and progress*. Routledge.

Miller, S. D., Hubble, M. A., & Chow, D. (2020). *Better results: Using deliberate practice to improve therapeutic effectiveness*. American Psychological Association.

Miller, S. D., Hubble, M. A., Chow, D. L., & Seidel, J. A. (2013). The outcome of psychotherapy: Yesterday, today, and tomorrow. *Psychotherapy, 50*(1), 88–97. https://doi.org/10.1037/a0031097

Natynczuk, S. (2014). Solution-focused practice as a useful addition to the concept of adventure therapy. *InterAction, 6*(1), 23–36.

Natynczuk, S. (2021). Co-adventuring for change: A solution-focused framework for "unspoken" therapy outdoors. *Relational Child and Youth Care Practice, 34*(4), 58–66.

Ratner, H., George, E., & Iveson, C. (2012). *Solution focused brief therapy: 100 key points and techniques*. Routledge.

Selekman, M. D. (1993). *Pathways to change: Brief therapy solutions with difficult adolescents* (1st ed.) Guildford Publishing.

Selekman, M. D. (2005). *Pathways to change: Brief therapy with difficult adolescents* (2nd ed.) Guilford Publishing.

Shennan, G. (2019). *Solution-focused practice: Effective communication to facilitate change* (2nd ed.) Red Globe Press.

Sparks, J., Duncan, B. L., & Miller, S. D. (2007). Common factors and the uncommon heroism of youth. *Psychotherapy in Australia, 13*(2), 34–43.

Tucker, A. R., Bettmann, J. E., Norton, C. L., & Comart, C. (2015). The role of transport use in adolescent wilderness treatment: Its relationship to readiness to change and outcomes. *Child & Youth Care Forum, 44*(5), 671–686. https://doi.org/10.1007/s10566-015-9301-6

Tucker, A. R., Combs, K. M., Bettmann, J. E., Chang, T. H., Graham, S., Hoag, M., & Tatum, C. (2018). Longitudinal outcomes for youth transported to wilderness therapy programs. *Research on Social Work Practice, 28*(4), 438–451. https://doi.org/10.1177%2F1049731516647486

Tucker, A. R., & Norton, C. L. (2013). The use of adventure therapy techniques by clinical social workers: Implications for practice and training. *Clinical Social Work Journal, 41*(4), 333–343. https://doi.org/10.1007/s10615-012-0411-4

Wampold, B. E., & Imel, Z. E. (2015). *The great psychotherapy debate: The evidence for what makes psychotherapy work* (2nd ed.) Routledge.

Weiner-Davis, M., de Shazer, S., & Gingerich, W. J. (1987). Building on pretreatment change to construct the therapeutic solution: An exploratory study. *Journal of Marital and Family Therapy, 13*(4), 359–363. https://doi.org/10.1111/j.1752-0606.1987.tb00717.x

6

Expedition Settings and Group Work

"When we sit down together, I know we are embarking on a journey to a destination that cannot be precisely specified and via routes that cannot be predetermined. I know that we will probably take some extraordinary scenic routes to these unknown destinations. I know that as we approach these destinations we will be stepping into other worlds of experience. And I know that the adventures to be had on these journeys are not about the confirmation of what is already known, but about expeditions into what is possible for people to know about their lives."

Michael White (2007, p. 4)

Much of this chapter relates to our experiences and observations from therapeutic expeditions. This model is informed from wilderness therapy experiences across the United States, Australia, Canada, the UK, Indonesia, and Norway. These expeditions typically involve traveling, possibly backpacking or canoeing, in a small group each day to set up a new campsite. Some of this will likely have a familiar ring for the experienced expedition-based practitioner. We hope you notice how a solution-focus can weave seamlessly throughout a multi-day expedition.

In the spirit of *adventurosity*, we agree with White (2007) that all therapy endeavors lead to uncertain destinations. We may be tempted to plan every minute of the expedition or lean on a problem-saturated narrative to justify why a certain person should attend. Building on previous chapters, the expedition is a container for people to witness and experience what is possible in their lives. Practitioners working in expedition settings embrace the unknown and work with each meaningful moment as it emerges.

Solution-focused events usually start with asking about people's preferred futures and their best hopes. This should be established early on. During the expedition, checking progress against best hopes should be part of regular

DOI: 10.4324/9781003217558-8

campfire sessions. This chapter analyzes how practitioners balance the role of therapist and outdoor guide, providing considerations for hosting useful expeditions. There is little literature about what the expedition-based practitioner actually does. We look forward to continued dialogue about what others have found useful in their work. The back half of this chapter will provide implications for those working with groups in the outdoors.

Background to Therapy Expeditions

In the United States, Russell and Hendee (2000) described four common types of wilderness therapy programs. These four models are:

1) **contained expedition** programs, where clients and the treatment team remain together on a wilderness expedition.
2) **continuous flow expedition** programs, where leaders, therapists, and clients rotate in and out of ongoing groups in the wilderness.
3) **base camp expedition** programs, which have structured base camps in natural environments and take expedition outings from the base.
4) **residential expedition** programs, which include emotional growth schools, residential treatment centers, Job Corps Centers, youth ranches, and other therapeutic designations that use wilderness and outdoor treatment as a tool to augment other services for resident clients.

(p. 3)

We remain vigilant to client choice and privilege people's perception of what is working and what is not. Those who attend our adventures should be prepared for what is happening and know when the expedition will conclude. While we believe solution-focused outdoor therapy can be implemented in long-term residential treatment and on continuous-flow wilderness therapy programs, that is not our focus here. We have already questioned the ethics of holding people against their will (Dobud, 2021), only granting their leave when they meet what practitioners believe are appropriate therapeutic goals, for example what DeMille and Montgomery (2017) described as therapist *gatekeeping* in OBH programs.

We take a close look at contained expeditions, where a group starts the adventure together, and completes it at the same time, where all adventurers begin with similar footing. As expedition leaders, we have certain roles to play. We monitor safety, therapeutic progress, and host what is sure to be a fun, exciting, and engaging experience, no matter the length of time.

Hosting an Outdoor Therapy Expedition

We use the following sections to examine how the mindset of hosting becomes essential in outdoor therapy expeditions. What we are not going to take is a deep dive into how one becomes a safe and competent expedition leader. As we stressed thus far, where your work takes place will have politics, policies, laws, guidelines, certifications, and mandates for running certain programs, each so specific we would not have space to examine them here. Make sure you get acquainted with relevant guidelines, permissions, and regulations. Remember, practitioners do not have to be constantly busy with therapy. The group will need time to process their experiences among themselves.

Being a Solution-Focused Expedition Leader

Therapeutic expedition leader is a tough role. You wear many metaphorical hats. In one moment, you are an adventure guide, reading a topographic map with a compass, and the next a caring psychotherapist. You will be a cook, survivalist, medic, logistic planner, risk management specialist, safety officer, teacher, facilitator, coach, guide, empath, and superhero all in one program, perhaps even all in one day.

Congruence and genuineness, those famous core conditions for therapeutic change (Rogers, 1957), are essential to expedition work. You are in center stage every moment and your co-adventurers will have you on strict observation. One of the greatest opportunities in outdoor therapy, and specifically on multi-day programs, is the rich amount of time you share with incredible people. Practitioners hear stories of trauma, inspiration, change, and dogged determination. For many therapy recipients, this amount of time with helping professionals feels drastically different to a weekly visit to a clinician's couch. This is a true shared experience. If it rains, it rains on all of you. You get to sit and watch a soaring eagle or sleep around a fire while gazing up at the billions of stars shining overhead, all together.

You may also be awoken after someone has a nightmare or wets the bed. Ask any experienced expedition leader about toileting stories, it is common. You may sit with a homesick child at two in the morning and share stories while they fall back asleep. You may be the recipient of a mouthful of threats or verbal attacks. Additionally, you and your leadership team may have a rupture in your relationship. Then, you will have to figure out how to repair your relationships at night, losing precious hours of sleep. To aid the reflection process while on expedition, Appendix J provides a guide to maintaining a solution-focus and avoiding problem-saturated discussions.

How you respond to all of these experiences will impact the experience of your co-adventurers. When constructing your team of practitioners, consider whose skill sets will complement your own. No practitioner can be created perfectly in your image. We two have managed successful outdoor therapy practices and appreciate that no employee will care about our programs as much as we do. We must allow them to be their best when we are out in the field. Otherwise, like disengaged therapy clients, they will not come back. We know expedition work has a high staff turnover. Let your teammates contribute their best selves. This way, they can be genuine and congruent with the co-adventurers too!

There will be times for formal group therapy work, such as having a talking circle around the fire, and more informal times, like during a canoe paddle down the river. We recommend viewing therapy as intertwined and seamless throughout the entire expedition, not something that only occurs at various structured times. You can always ask solution-focused questions whenever you see fit. Co-adventurers will feel safe to talk at the most unusual times and places.

Imagine a 15-year-old referred to your expedition for behavior issues in school. The student was known for kicking chairs, swearing at teachers, and bullying other students. During a canoe expedition, he takes a turn steering from the back of the boat. The other participant in the front is not a confident paddler and you notice this participant exhibiting patience, speaking calmly, and helping the other participant feel more comfortable. After landing a high five, you say: "I have seen a lot of people get really frustrated paddling with other people! That was amazing. You were so patient and helpful. How did you do that?"

"I don't know," he responds.

"Is that different than usual?" you ask.

"Yes, it is. I would just get up, call him a name, and walk away." The client has provided a rich experience of success and mastery and described an exception to the problem that landed him on your expedition. Before reading on, think about what you would say or ask to help your co-adventurer construct further meaning from this experience towards their preferred future. Here are some ideas that we have:

- Do you have a name for the kind of "patience" you just exhibited?
- If you were able to demonstrate this same level of patience in the classroom, what would your teachers notice?
- What difference do you think that level of patience will make at home?
- If you were going to be this kind of focused for the remainder of the expedition, what would we notice from you?

If you save "therapy" time for specific moments, penciled into a predetermined schedule, you might miss the opportunity for helping participants to consolidate the gains they have made at various times. Still, it is not a bad idea to hold a structured reflection session around the fire, or to ask specific group therapy questions, but stay focused on observing these moments of competence, success, and mastery in the moment. In the busyness of a day on expedition, you do not want to lose the opportunity to examine these successes with solution-focused questioning. Think hard about the best time to ask questions so the vital observation is not ruined in that precious moment.

The First Day

Your participants arrive and they are ready to go. Maybe you outfit them with all the gear they need or provide a packing list so they show up kitted out ready to explore. The first day can tend to be overly administrative, talking about group rules, safety, and a plethora of policies. It can be easy to lose focus on engagement, the therapeutic relationship, and the purpose for the program. If you have a team of outdoor guides, choose one to teach various skills, like setting up a shelter or packing a backpack appropriately. This way, you can take care to observe the group, listen attentively, and use your solution-focused skills to elicit the best hopes of your co-adventurers.

Mastering all the skills required for successful expeditioning will be overwhelming to many of your unprepared participants. If they were involuntarily sent to you, or court ordered, they may feel certain there will be no benefit of their attendance. Practitioners should not avoid these truths. If this is your client's reality, collaborate and partner with their view of the world. This is one way we express empathy for their situation.

Take things slow on the first day. If you have a week or longer together, the participants have ample time to master various skills and obtain self-sufficiency. Many will have traveled some distance to reach a remote wilderness area and could be tired, hungry, anxious, or scared. Pick one skill you find most important for Day 1, such as setting up their tent and sleeping area, and focus the rest of your efforts on being a good host and eliciting best hopes.

We have observed very abrupt, distressing starts to programs. While some prefer a more prescriptive approach to guiding, with long instructions on the preferred means for rolling, or stuffing a sleeping bag into its bag, we must not forget our role as *host*. Day 1 may involve showing the participants how to set up a shelter or tent, and we make sure everyone is successful in doing so. Some will learn best by working it out themselves, while others may need to observe you erecting a tent multiple times. Others prefer diagrams. It is a good idea to cater to all of these learning preferences, when possible (Selekman, 2005).

When I (Stephan) work with school groups on expeditions, we usually meet in the afternoon at a public campsite. There, co-adventurers can unwind, learn how to put up their tents, and discover the items they, or someone they have designated to pack, have forgotten. I bring spare sleeping bags, tents, stoves, rain jackets, thermal clothing, and so on. Once on Axel-Heiberg Island, I asked a young person where their waterproofs were. "It wasn't raining in Montreal, so I didn't think I needed them" was the answer. Expect the unexpected. We distributed the food for the trip, including fresh vegetables and dried pulses for that night's stew. Occasionally, I come across people who have never peeled a root vegetable or chopped an onion. Responsibility for self-rationing food is delegated as part of the experiential learning from the expedition.

Once a young man, a strong character, decided someone else in his group would carry his food. He was surprised that two days into a four-day mountain walk, the others had eaten a portion of his food. The learning here was priceless. I always carry emergency food and a spare meal or two and am willing to lend a hand when things get a little too challenging. One morning, a co-adventurer stood in the drizzle waiting for his Trangia stove to self-assemble. This is a good time to gently step in to help with kindness.

We find it useful to model all of the skills participants will learn, such as sparking a fire with a flint and steel, or cooking over the fire, washing up, and getting everything inside a rucksack. This will arouse your participants' curiosity, one of our additional Crucial C's (Lew & Bettern, 1996). By day two or three, you will have participants asking if you can show them how to light the fire or offering to help with cooking dinner. We tell our participants early on that all we want is for them to feel comfortable and safe in the group. The team of practitioners might cook all meals early on and host wondrous dinner parties around the campfire or stove. Share stories around the fire, ask questions about when your co-adventurers are at their best, and make dinner time a highlight of the program. No one should eat alone.

It is common for participants to be anxious about sleeping early in the process. For your younger participants, this may be the furthest they have been from their parents, and the first time sleeping outdoors. Some may be used to falling asleep with the television on or scrolling on their phone. We have found it useful to bring a book, such as *The Knight in Rusty Armor* (Fisher, 1987), to read each night around the fire. At the start, some participants may not enjoy the reading but most, if not all, will enjoy a fun and lighthearted story with impeccable metaphors for therapeutic expedition work. Let the participants know where you are sleeping and that they can wake you for anything. We have found it useful to keep a cheap solar light near our shelter so participants can find us if disoriented in the dark.

When participants do begin the journey in the dark to their sleeping bags, take time to go visit each of them before they doze off. Make sure all their gear is safely stored so they will not get wet, put away any loose food, and ask if they have any questions about the plan for tomorrow. Make fine adjustments to their tents, to the cords and pegs, put their boots under the fly-sheet, to show you are looking out for them. Point out when you noticed them at their best and communicate your excitement for the next day's adventure.

Agreeing on Expectations and Establishing Boundaries

A therapeutic expedition requires a plan of action. What food will you provide? What rituals will you have for eating? Which non-negotiable ground rules will you set to ensure group cohesion and safety? Think about swearing, intimacy, mobile phone use, bedtimes, wake up times, how far a participant can journey from the group, where the toileting area is, where to get water, how far apart the tents should be, how you keep a look out for dangerous animals, and all of the considerations you will make. Here, we are presenting the customs we find useful in our expedition work. This may provide an idea as to what our programs look like in action.

Setting clear boundaries and expectations is important in group work, but some programs blow this far out of proportion. Outdoor therapy practitioners should reflect on their motivation to set different rules or expectations: who is doing the learning and whose life is being made easier with these rules? Write a list of what you think is most important and circle what you refer to as the *non-negotiables*. For us, swearing is not a problem, though it can quickly get out of hand. What difference does it make if we start a program with, "No swearing on this trip or there will be consequences," versus

> "Listen, swearing is part of everyday life. If we stub our toe, we might yell 'Shit!' That is fine, but sometimes it gets out of hand where it feels like swearing is every third word coming out of our mouths, including my own. If that happens, we'll work together to see what agreements we can make, cool?"

One approach invites resistance, the other collaboration. Never make threats, they are not therapeutic, and young people are usually expert at boundary testing and confrontation. This also gives you time to prioritize the non-negotiable rules and deal with the smaller stuff as your alliance improves. Swearing is much easier to work on within an established relationship.

What are non-negotiables? For us, they are quite simple. Be kind to each other, take care of yourself, your belongings, and others, protect the environments we travel on, and no racism, sexism, or bigotry. Maybe not *that* simple. Only one of these agreements comes with a "no" at the start of it. Ask the participants for other ideas for what could make the expedition experience more enjoyable and beneficial. If the group's rules are insufficient, we might prompt thinking by asking "what if" questions. Rules are easier to apply if negotiated.

We will not get into how to set boundaries and expectations further but wish to provide a word of caution. We have witnessed expedition programs where clients are expected to memorize a list of rules and expectations ranging from giving their boots to their field guides at night to prevent runaways, no talking to fellow co-adventurers without the presence of a staff member and calling out their name or assigned number while going to the toilet, signaling to the field staff where they are located (Dobud, 2020). We are therapeutic practitioners, not prison guards. Punitive expeditions are not what we do. Stay focused on the purpose of the program and everyone's best hopes.

Revisit some of the stances we examined in Chapter 4. We hope that chapter is useful for not only therapeutically oriented practitioners, but educators and recreation specialists. While discussing rules and expectations of co-adventurers may seem far afield from our solution-focused approach, we rely on Mitten's (1994) feminist critique of adventure therapy ethics for sound advice. Outdoor leaders who expect long lists of rules and expectations help to:

> maintain the status quo in our patriarchal society and gives both the leaders and the group a great deal of control over behavior. Given the power that leaders have in this situation, clients are undoubtedly, to a certain extent, compliant. This leaves little room for individual needs. These are the very needs that were overlooked that helped the clients become dysfunctional.
>
> (p. 66)

The more control a group leader exerts over a client, the more we seek the need for *compliance*, which is not a therapeutic outcome. We urge line managers and clinical directors to reconsider the rules they set. Resistance is interactional. It emerges from the relationship and is not a characteristic trait or a quality of a person's personality. If you sense what may be "resistance," better align your work with the client's preferences. Focus on each person's dignity and best hopes for their future. Reflect on people's right to experience and how we can privilege their self-determination. It is their adventure, not ours.

When working with a team of expedition staff, it is imperative to prepare for the adventure by getting to know each other and working out what you will do when things go wrong. What is the game plan when an expectation is not met, or a boundary crossed? If one of the staff feels frustrated or triggered by a participant's behavior, how will the other staff step up to help? These considerations are important when facilitating a journey.

Journeying

Most expedition programs are characterized by traveling each day to a new campsite. You might be hiking, canoeing, sailing, or any other form of travel. Some overnight programs stay at a base camp and go on daily adventures. No matter the form of travel, this section examines some solution-focused considerations for day-to-day travel while in the field.

Considering various levels of engagement is important during an expedition. There is an unstated expectation that everyone can keep up and stay together. Participants with varying capabilities may become quickly demoralized if they fall behind or struggle through a particular journey. Hiking with a backpack can be grueling, paddling a canoe frustrating. The focus on success and mastery and the climate of competence are important to consider throughout the day. The team should continue to engage participants in interesting discussion, especially in the early days as participants become accustomed to the daily adventures and routines.

The journey is an opportunity for the practitioner to model their genuineness. If your feet are sore or your back hurts, it is okay to communicate that. Let your co-adventurers see the real you. Point out interesting plants, fauna, geomorphology, and archeology; watch the weather forming on the horizon. Arouse curiosity. Take frequent breaks to allow for rest and relaxation, and to replenish energy with trail mix. Expeditions should be fun and exciting, not a slog or endurance battle. As one participant put it, "hiking did not make me contemplate my sins" (Dobud, 2020). The therapeutic aspects come from the practitioner's work in asking questions to construct therapeutic meaning.

As a host inviting participants to engage actively in what many may find taxing, practitioners should make extra effort to bring fun, curiosity, and adventurosity into the experience. We remind our reader that these experiences are void of therapeutic value until co-adventurers place meaning on them. We do so similarly when organizing food and eating together around a fire.

Food

The fire is crackling. People have kicked off their hiking boots. Stomachs are growling after a long day of trekking or paddling. Dinner time around the campfire is what our experience has shown to be some of the most beneficial times during an expedition. That said, we have witnessed outdoor programs to also use mealtime as a time for restriction or control of people's experiences. For example, some wilderness therapy programs require participants to complete a certain number of daily tasks, such as bow drilling a fire, in order to enjoy a hot meal, one warmed over a fire. Creating a hierarchy in the group invites opposition. We, instead, view the sharing of a meal around the campfire as a sacred time for promoting engagement. Your co-adventurers are given yet another chance to witness the real, genuine you, and work together.

Organizing a group shelter so everyone can sit out of the weather is ideal, though not always possible. Sometimes co-adventurers are in small groups and share a stove and food. This is especially true of winter expeditions and times of rainy weather when people might prefer to hunker down as soon as it gets cold and dark.

Focusing on host leadership (McKergow & Pugliese, 2019) is a good place to start. From the early days of an expedition ensure participants are warm, safe, and well-fed. Modeling host leadership demonstrates positive regard and empathy for co-adventurers (Natynczuk, 2019). We like to prepare meals in front of the participants while asking engaging questions, much like your cheesy dinner party conversation starters. Participants may ask what they can help with, much like we would as a guest in a close friend's home. Put them to work. Give group members an onion to chop or a can of beans to drain. This will provide a moment of success and mastery and invites further quality participation in the experience. Little things matter.

As participants get to know each other, you will spend less time in the spotlight during mealtime. Early on, however, you will likely prepare dinner while engaging in conversation. Mention how much you enjoy sharing meals with great people. Discuss why you chose the food you have. If it is possible, do the expedition food shopping with co-adventurers. The bigger the process for preparing the meal, like chopping onions, soaking dehydrated beans, or kneading a damper, the better. This gives you time to connect with participants while expressing care.

For some, the food an outdoor therapy program caters is the most nutritional diet they have consumed in some time. While extended expeditions require careful planning around the sustainability of produce and perishable goods, we do argue for bringing in the most wholesome ingredients possible. We avoid pre-packaged ready meals and prefer meals that require some preparation and little waste. Plastic and cans can quickly add up so it is important to consider how waste will be dealt with to best leave no trace.

Teaching Skills

Learning to roll a sleeping bag, pack a rucksack, spark a fire, sleep in the dirt, tie specific knots, navigate with a map and compass, poop in the woods, or paddle a canoe is a lot. Add to this navigating the social dynamics of a group and our therapeutic programs can be quite overwhelming! We avoid using skills as behavior modification or preventing participants from progressing in a program. Additionally, because success and mastery are important to the climate of competence, we adapt and amend based on a co-adventurer's strengths and capabilities. For example, one participant may find the physical exertion related to paddling a canoe more difficult than the next. Assuming both need to learn the skill homogenizes those we work with, which we avoid at all costs.

Maintaining the experiential framework, solution-focused practitioners refrain from viewing skills and techniques as experiential. Many people paddle canoes, rock climb, and spark fires without receiving any therapeutic value. In fact, most people rock climb for the first time in their lives at a six-year-old friend's birthday party at the climbing gym. What gives these activities therapeutic value is the meaning the participant freely constructs about the experience. Remaining diligent in people's best hopes will help to reduce the tendency to appropriate therapeutic meaning to skills.

That said, if we are required to teach a number of skills, for safety and educational purposes, take it slow. Ideally teach skills in context, and just before they are needed. Make sure to scaffold the tasks based on what feels most important. Fixating on the skills we teach invites compliance. The more practitioners underscore the importance of outdoor skills, the more co-adventurers stress about them. Thus, their experience is about memorizing skills and less about their best hopes or the reasons they came to therapy.

People learn in different ways. We should cater to the strengths and capabilities of those we work with. We avoid overcomplicating what we teach and abstain from homogenizing skills across all group members where possible. If one participant gets a kick from fire making, and another when navigating, we tailor the expedition to these preferences. The door is open for participants to engage in any activity they wish to do more of and avoid what they have tried and did not find meaningful.

Postcards from Home

When I (Will) entered the field of wilderness therapy, I was a young field guide with no clinical training really excited about working outdoors with adolescents who seemed to experience similar teenager challenges I had. While I was an experienced *therapy veteran* (Duncan et al., 1997), as someone who sat on many therapist couches during my youth, I was positively thrilled by working with therapeutic intent out of doors. I knew early on this was what I wanted to do. That said, there were many practices in my early years of American wilderness therapy I look back on with concern. One of these was the *Impact Letter*.

According to Tucker et al. (2016), the impact letter is a commonly used intervention in wilderness therapy. The letters are used for:

> describing how the parent's life has been affected by the child's be-havior, writing in direct frank language, but avoiding hostility and blaming. Family therapists may teach parents to repackage the mes-sage in a way that it is easier for their child to listen and understand their experience ... The child then reads the letter to his or her peers around a campfire at night.
>
> (pp. 35–36)

To be honest, I was initially moved watching young people read these let-ters. I thought this was a provoking process. I have seen participants break down into tears and feel compelled to reflect on their decisions and how they have impacted those closest to them. That said, there were equally as many participants declaring, "This is bullshit! This is a fake version of my parents. Why aren't they addressing how my dad hit and tackled me just the other week?" When building my own practice, I experienced a crisis in faith. Should I invite parents and clients to write to each other throughout our expeditions, or just let it go?

I decided to turn the process on its head and go with a solution-focus. On the fourth day of our expedition, when participants spark their own fires, I bring the participants their first letter from home. They are not co-erced into reading it aloud and the vibe of the letter is drastically different. Here is the prompt we provide the parents:

> "It is time for you to email your first letter that we will process with your child. This letter is designed to spark some new communication in the family and provide more time for reflection. It is a powerful day in the field as your child will learn how to spark a fire with no matches or lighters and will sit with the field staff to present the letter.
>
> We ask for this letter to arrive before 9am on Day 4. If you have been following this workbook, that is tomorrow morning. We've outlined some thoughts for this letter below."

1) Ask about what your child has been doing. Questions about food, the staff, and the skills they've learned are good options.
2) Talk about the work you have been doing. What have you learned through True North's parent program so far? What has been most important to you?
3) Talk about your "best hopes" for participating in this program. This is not a time to lecture. Shame is the last feeling we want as it can be demoralizing. Think about what the two of you would be doing together if your best hopes materialized.

4) End with niceties. Let your child know they are valued and loved.
5) Remember, True North Expeditions is a "Where To" program and hope is required for a future focus. The goal of this letter is to build hope for a more positive future. One where the problems that brought you to True North are no longer present.

Of course, this is quite a prescribed template, but remember, the problem narrative that sees someone on our expeditions is often laden with Killer D's (Duncan, 2014). Adolescents can feel they are in trouble when sent on an expedition. By inviting the parents and adolescents to explore their preferred future, we shift that narrative. We invite our co-adventurers to sit by their fire and write a reply. If they need longer to digest, that is fine.

Since we have worked with adolescents for the majority of our careers, we do describe more implications for working with parents in the following chapter. That said, not all of you will work with young people. If letter writing feels like something you would like to implement in this work, consider a solution-focus. More therapeutic experiments like these are available in the field manual and examined in the next chapter.

In contrast, I (Stephan) tend not to use letters from parents. I have seen the distress and public humiliation of young people not getting a letter when their peers have. We can use third person perspectives to talk about what parents and carers, siblings and friends might notice when things between them are better.

Journaling

There is nothing wrong allocating specific time for participants to write in a journal and consolidate their reflections on the outdoor therapy expeditions. That said, prescribing such a task can backfire. Be mindful of forcing your co-adventurers to spend specific amounts of time reflecting on their experience through a journal. Some will place little to no meaning on the practice, and we have worked with organizations where daily journaling is absolute. If your program uses daily writing as a time for reflection, there is no reason not to incorporate solution-focused questions in your journal prompts. Appendix I in the field manual includes possible journaling prompts you can utilize.

Journaling is a therapeutic experiment participants use to reflect on their experiences and consolidate gains (Selekman & Beyebach, 2014). Similarly, paper and pen can be used for a range of art therapy techniques.

A word of caution about journaling, however, is that some clients simply will not care. We should avoid overemphasizing the prescription of specific interventions, like journaling. If a co-adventurer loves journaling and really engages with the process, do more of it. If they do not, let it go and search for a more appealing activity to aid their reflection. In our work and research, we have witnessed programs use journaling to prohibit participants from advancing in the program. Under no circumstance do we use therapeutic initiatives for gatekeeping as this will lead to resistance or compliance with the prescribed tasks (Mitten, 1994), not therapeutic outcomes.

Aiding the Transfer of Learning

Closing an expedition should be a humanizing experience. While it may be tempting to avoid discussions about what comes next in a co-adventurer's life, we have found it necessary to focus as much on building group cohesion and a climate of competence as closing the group. One strategy is to move on from the outdoor environment and celebrate the experience in a different setting. A group may move from the rural and remote outdoor setting to a location closer to home. As the program facilitators adopt a secondary role, co-adventurers experientially enact aspects of their preferred future in a new environment, one less structured than the contained expedition.

The more opportunities participants have to experience and notice the changes they described while on expedition, the better. The transfer of learning occurs when people apply what they learnt on expedition to a new setting (Perkins & Salomon, 1992). Pilots rehearse with a simulator so incidents in the cockpit do not catch them by surprise. Army soldiers practice scenarios and drills so the stress of a real-life combat situation does not impact decision making and tactics. These two professions are historically regarded as best for the transfer of learning. We have a lot to learn from these fields when change occurs outside of a person's community environment.

As an expedition closes, outdoor solution-focused practitioners provide ongoing moments to live their climate of competence in new settings. For example, if the expedition leaders have scheduled for the final three nights of the experience to take place in a cabin closer to the participants' home, the practitioner can ask what participants would notice about themselves, or each other, if they were continuing to be at their best in the new setting. Over those final days, use these moments to direct people's lived experience to life after the expedition. Questions one may ask include:

- I noticed today you offered to help cook for the group. If you did this upon returning home, what would your parents notice? What difference would this make?
- What will be the first thing you (or key stakeholder) will notice upon you returning home to suggest this expedition was particularly meaningful for you?
- What difference has this expedition made for you?
- If I checked in with you in a week's time, what improvements would you like to tell me about?
- I saw you really focused during our expedition. Who in your life will be the first person to notice if you enact this more at home?
- What have you gained from this experience?
- What do you think you did to keep going during this expedition? What difference could that make when you return home?

To aid the transfer of learning, practitioners ask future-focused questions related to the success and mastery of their co-adventurers' experience. When noticing people adventuring at their best, questions are asked to invite clients to suppose how life would be different if they transferred this experience to life after the program. To construct more solutions, ask what key stakeholders, such as the parole officer, parent, or spouse, would notice when these changes materialize.

Aftercare and Follow-Up

Co-adventurers have typically exercised daily, improved their sleep routine, enjoyed a balanced diet, and got to engage for some time with supportive people. They are feeling great. Upon returning home, however, there are setbacks. The ups and downs of everyday life come storming back, and quite possibly the solutions they discovered on expedition are more difficult to enact.

I (Will) spent the beginning of my career working on any wilderness therapy programs that would take me. Our participants remained on these programs for an average of 90 days and many transitioned to ongoing residential treatment or therapeutic boarding schools, increasing the amount of time they remained away from home. In 2006, I was invited by my mentor Brooke Brody to start an aftercare program for these young people returning home. I learnt very quickly that implementing the changes made away from home was difficult. What seemed important during their time away seemed to matter less at home. We focused our work on bringing wilderness therapy home.

When following up with co-adventurers, we maintain our ethic to leave no trace in our clients' lives (Natynczuk & Dobud, 2021). Let them know we are free for a phone call or an individual adventure whenever they want. We do not prescribe follow-up activities but advise that some have benefited from them and others have found them unnecessary. The open-door policy described in the previous chapter applies when expeditions close.

It may be tempting to refer a person for ongoing therapy thinking this will help maintain progress. This can demoralize people. In a perfect world, participants have experienced days on end successfully expeditioning in wild environments building exceptional evidence of their best self. The referral to ongoing therapy forces them to start a new therapeutic relationship. However, the new practitioner may ignore the gains experienced during the expedition. A problem-focused practitioner may disregard the outdoor therapy experience, believe their type of therapy is more impactful than another, or suppose a new assessment of the client's Killer D's is required.

When co-adventurers call for a tune up session or wish to continue adventuring with you after the expedition, we follow their lead and organize our sessions similar to how we described previously, beginning with asking about what has been better and their best hopes for the session. We may invite reflection about the expedition and what meaning continues to be relevant in the person's life.

Aftercare and follow-up are typically recommended by practitioners, not clients. We remain diligent to client choice and their best hopes. If they feel ongoing support would be useful, we recommend practitioners in their community, provide outdoor therapy ourselves, or offer virtual sessions via phone or video conferencing. More therapy is indicated when it is part of a client's best hopes. That said, do not be a stranger. You have spent multiple days outdoors, shared meals and many laughs. Clients got to see the real you. If we ghost them, this may rupture the real relationship they perceived and deteriorate the meaning constructed during the expedition.

Solution-Focused Group Work Outdoors

We have noticed many outdoor group therapy approaches include a time for the group members to sit, typically in a circle, for what may look like "typical" group therapy. This can be a good time for reflecting on the day, consolidating, or exploring times during the day's adventure when people experienced success, mastery, or exceptions. What we hope to stress in this section is that you can maintain a solution-focus during these groups, preserving emotional and psychological safety and avoiding retraumatizing your participants with problem-saturated discussions (Gass et al., 2012). Recall the impact letter described earlier in this chapter, a letter typically read aloud around the fire with other participants seated in a circle. This problem-focused approach is irreconcilable with our solution-focused stance.

You can use simple solution-focused activities or pick a theme for the group, for example, "Who has been your greatest advocate? What have they done?" These groups can be brief and unstructured (Bannink, 2010). Allow space for casual conversation. You may conduct an experiential activity and use solution-focused questions to debrief the scenario. Participants can work in small groups discussing your solution-focused questions among themselves. You might start with suggesting they make a list of all the things they were pleased to notice today and to share these in their small groups.

In a rural and remote school, we facilitated an activity with a group of 15 adolescents. We split them into three groups and gave each a survival scenario. One, for example, was a desert island scenario and another was being lost in the remote Australian bush while four-wheel driving. In the scenario, the participants are required to choose from a list of 20 items which five items are most important for their survival. The group constructs a plan of action using these items. After finding consensus about their plan, we ask what skills and mindset their group would need to flourish in this scenario. When participants describe leadership or communication skills, being cooperative, and helping each other, we treated these as moments of imagined mastery and asked what they would notice if they did this in real life. To close the group, we asked participants to describe what would be the first thing they would notice after this group to indicate they are making this happen.

This is one example of how a solution-focus can impact group work. The participants cooperated with each other and used an experiential activity to construct solutions. The co-adventurers learnt from each other's ideas and applied the meaning made from the activity to life outside the group. In the spirit of co-adventuring, the teachers and group leaders were active participants in the group, demonstrating their authentic selves to the students.

Conclusion

Solution-focused practice lends itself to outdoor therapy expeditions and group work. When facilitating experiences of success and mastery, practitioners use future-focused questions to help co-adventurers place meaning on the unique solutions they discovered. The solution-focused group leader remains vigilant in being a good host. In this chapter, we discussed many ideas for running outdoor therapy expeditions and briefly explored some considerations for group work.

The following chapter examines how we can work with referrers and parents as allies for change. Part III of this book, which follows after the next chapter, considers ways for putting all of this work together, beginning with supervision, feedback-informed treatment, and avoiding burnout.

References

Bannink, F. (2010). *1001 solution-focused questions: Handbook for solution-focused interviewing.* W. W. Norton & Co.

DeMille, S. M., & Montgomery, M. J. (2017). A case study of narrative family therapy in an outdoor treatment program with a struggling adolescent. In J. D. Christenson & A. N. Merritts (Eds.), *Family Therapy with Adolescents in Residential Treatment* (pp. 29–48). Springer. https://doi.org/10.1007/978-3-319-51747-6_3

Dobud, W. W. (2020). *Experiences of adventure therapy: A narrative inquiry* [Doctoral Dissertation]. Charles Sturt University.

Dobud, W. W. (2021). Experiences of secure transport in outdoor behavioral healthcare: A narrative inquiry. *Qualitative Social Work.* https://doi.org/10.1177%2F14733250211020088

Duncan, B. L. (2014). *On becoming a better therapist: Evidence-based practice one client at a time.* American Psychological Association.

Duncan, B. L., Hubble, M. A., & Miller, S. D. (1997). *Psychotherapy with "impossible" cases: The efficient treatment of therapy veterans.* W. W. Norton & Co.

Fisher, R. (1987). *The knight in rusty armor.* Wilshire Book Company.

Gass, M. A., Gillis, H. L., & Russell, K. C. (2012). *Adventure therapy: Theory, research, and practice*. Routledge.

Lew, A., & Bettern, B. L. (1996). *A parent's guide to understanding and motivating children*. Connexions Press.

McKergow, M., & Pugliese, P. (Eds.) (2019). *The host leadership field book: Building engagement for performance and results*. Solution Books.

Mitten, D. (1994). Ethical considerations in adventure therapy: A feminist critique. *Women & Therapy, 15*(3–4), 55–84. https://doi.org/10.1300/J015v15n03_06

Natynczuk, S. (2019). Host leadership in outdoor, bush, wilderness and adventure therapy in M. McKergow and P. Pugliese (Eds.), *The host leadership field book: Building engagement for performance and results* (pp. 42–52). Solution Books.

Natynczuk, S., & Dobud, W. W. (2021). Leave no trace, willful unknowing, and implications from the ethics of sustainability for solution-focused practice outdoors. *Journal of Solution Focused Practices, 5*(2), 7.

Perkins, D. N., & Salomon, G. (1992). Transfer of learning. *International Encyclopedia of Education, 2*, 6452–6457.

Rogers, C. R. (1957). The necessary and sufficient conditions of therapeutic personality change. *Journal of Consulting Psychology, 21*(2), 95–103. https://doi.org/10.1037/h0045357

Russell, K. C., & Hendee, J. C. (2000). *Outdoor behavioral healthcare: Definitions, common practice, expected outcomes, and a nationwide survey of programs*. Technical Report #26, Moscow, Idaho. Idaho Forest, Wildlife and Range Experiment Station.

Selekman, M. D. (2005). *Pathways to change: Brief therapy with difficult adolescents* (2nd ed.) Guilford Publishing.

Selekman, M. D., & Beyebach, M. (2014). *Changing self-destructive habits: Pathways to solutions with couples and families*. Routledge.

Tucker, A. R., Widmer, M. A., Faddis, T., & Randolph, B. (2016). Family therapy in outdoor behavioral healthcare: Current practices and future possibilities. *Contemporary Family Therapy, 38*, 32–42. https://doi.org/10.1007/s10591-015-9370-6

White, M. K. (2007). *Maps of narrative practice*. W. W. Norton & Company.

7
Working with Parents and Referrers

"There are three ways of trying to win the young. There is persuasion, there is compulsion, and there is attraction. You can preach at them: that is a hook without a worm. You can say, You must volunteer, and that is of the devil. You can tell them, You are needed. That appeal hardly ever fails."

Kurt Hahn (in Gookin, 2012, n.p.)

"Meet the parents and meet the problem" (Gass et al., 2012, p. 62). We have heard this sentiment from many therapeutic practitioners working with young people. Indeed, there are probably over 100 people we could add to the phrase if we adopted this viewpoint. Meet the school, meet the bully, meet the negative influencing substance using peers, meet the problem. The list goes on with its complexity of connections and assumption-based blame.

After running my (Will) first expedition with True North Expeditions, Inc. with just three adolescent male participants, I was called to a school meeting. I had recently left my job at a large non-profit working with Indigenous young people and refugees from Syria and Sudan, saved a bit of money, bought ten sleeping bags and ten backpacks, figured out how to get insurance, and managed to find three young men and an outdoor educator to come on our first program. The meeting was with a 16-year-old participant named Jake, his school principal, school counselor, and the head of his year. His single mother was overseas and asked if I would attend.

As I walked into the school, I sensed a different version of the kid I had just spent the previous two weeks adventuring with in the outback. His hair was in his face, his gaze firmly planted at the ground. The principal addressed me, not Jake. "First off, we are glad Jake had such a good time on camp with you," I sensed his sarcasm. "But in the last two weeks, we have received 18 behavioral incidents written up in our system by the teachers." I felt like a

DOI: 10.4324/9781003217558-9

failure. I had left my job, built a small practice, earned the trust of parents to take their children on an adventure, tried to market myself to schools in the local area, and this was the feedback I received. I felt pushed into a corner.

Not knowing exactly what to say, I asked a pretty basic question. "Can I get an idea of what types of things have been happening?"

The principal shuffled the papers in front of him. "I don't think we need to unpack each incident. That would not be an appropriate use of our time." I intervened. "Well, as the social worker hired to…" Looking back, I realize the power struggle I was involved in.

And so, the principal began. "On March 22nd at 1:32pm, Jake received a complaint for uniform violation. On March 22nd at 2:55pm, Jake received a complaint for uniform violation. On March 23rd at 9:16am, Jake received a complaint for uniform violation." I looked at Jake. He looked at me and shrugged his shoulders letting out a small chuckle. I was sitting in a meeting with professionals talking about a student's clothing. I could not believe it. The good news, however, is that Jake's story took such a drastic and unexpected solution-focused turn.

Jake hung in with school for another few weeks before electing to drop out. Definitely not my preferred outcome or his mother's. He traveled interstate to work on a mountain as a snowboard instructor. Within a year, he began working in the United States and Canada. Two years later, he was one of the most sought-after youth snowboarding coaches in all of Australia, and a surprise to many – the Australian snowboarding team is good, *really* good. In 2019, he had taken over 40 flights for snowboarding competitions and training all over the world. Surprisingly, years later that same principal asked if he could showcase Jake as an alumnus in the school newspaper. Jake never graduated, though he has begun studying solution-focused brief therapy with hopes to implement more of this approach in his coaching. Remember, I was called into a meeting to discuss school uniforms.

Working with parents, schools, and other referrers adds an extra wrinkle to our work. Clearly in this case example, I was stuck in a problem-focused mindset, rather than taking the solution-focused lead and inviting discussion about everyone's best hopes on where we were headed and what we would notice if we were going in the right direction. In this chapter, we discuss our approach to this work. Included are "homework assignments," journal prompts, and specific questions we can ask in order to help our external parties adopt a solution, future, and hopeful focus. It is not meet the problem. It is meet the resource.

Who is the *Client*?

Often referrals come with a request for something similar to "Can you sort the lad out? He's such a disruptor of lessons." Being complicit with such a request we feel is solution-forced, as we would be working for some other person's interests. Not those of our client. I (Stephan) remember one case where a school was eager to prove no one could work with someone only to make this particular young person more easily permanently excluded from the school. This, I only learnt much later. Meanwhile, I engaged the student and provided evidence for many aspects of their good character and capabilities.

The client is the one in the room with us, the one at the other end of the phone, or the one on the video call, the one we are spending time with working for their best hopes. We can ask parents solution-focused questions, such as "If your child attends our program, what should we make sure does not change?" This asks what they, the parents, want their child to keep doing. We can, of course, ask such a question directly. We might invite them to let us know what they will notice indicating our work is impactful and helpful, subsequently asking what the client will notice about themselves illustrating they are moving in the best direction for their own hopes to be realized. We cannot be any more client-focused than asking what they want, and how they will know when they are moving towards it.

In this chapter, we present some of the solution-focused assumptions we take when working with families. This begins with how we approach our first contact with a young person's family members. We describe techniques for helping those invested in the adolescent's wellbeing to help be a witness to change and to consolidate the gains made during therapy. The chapter concludes with a brief illustration of some of the journaling or homework assignments we might provide parents and what to do if things go off the rails.

Working with Parents

When working with young people, parents are often the first point of contact. They are front and center stage witnesses to their child's deteriorating wellbeing, a decline frequently translated into concerns about problem behaviors, like self-harming or substance use. Of course, we must validate their concerns and listen attentively to the problem narrative. Remain cautious, however, not to adopt the problem-laden focus of the referral. Our focus is on what works and the difference more of it will make to the client's life.

When meeting with parents, we ask "How can we help?" This usually leads to an unpacking of how difficult things have been in the home. Take this seriously and listen attentively for exceptions. We will address how we can help work with parents to validate all their attempts to support their child throughout the following sections.

If a parent makes the effort to contact you, they might be nervous, maybe frustrated, anxious, scared, or embarrassed, or all of those. Recognize how demoralized they could be, how unsupported they might feel, and attempt to tune in with them. Though everyone may have contributed to the problem as they see it, avoid communicating blame or judgment. These phone calls can take time, and make sure to hear what the parent wants to communicate. Use reflective statements to convey empathy and do not push the conversation towards the client's engagement or offer advice. If you move too fast, you risk becoming solution-forced, which may leave the parent feeling demoralized and further frustrated, and leaves you in a tricky situation professionally.

During any initial consultation, we remind parents that therapy works, indoors or out, and that we should see benefit sooner, rather than later. We remind parents that *engagement* is our responsibility, not the child's. We are their hosts. To position parents as witnesses to change, we equip them with the evidence. If young people drop out of care, it is often due to a rupture in the therapeutic alliance; the young person needs to feel heard and understood. If parents do not see benefit from the therapy, they become less likely to bring their adolescent to the service. Thus, we need to know if they are satisfied by our work. Our clients are guests in the host approach, expecting some kind of preferred future. We position them as a witness of outcome. What will they notice if the work goes well for the client? These steps can not only validate the parents' experience of seeking help, or previous therapy failures. They also empower them to search for what is working and let us know when something is not.

After equipping parents with the available evidence, we ask a similar question to when we meet young clients for the first time: "How would you know our service has been useful?" or "How would you know that spending time with us has been a good use of your time?" We let parents know that we are interested in a "where to" answer to this question; not "where from." While this sounds like an argument of semantics, this is important. We avoid a future narrative of what will be absent. For example, fewer arguments at home or reductions in problematic behavior are of little interest to us. Likewise, simplistic answers about improved school attendance or happiness are only starting points. We follow these common responses with what parents will *notice* when their preferred future begins unfolding, and thus how they know we are moving in the preferred direction for the young person.

Being an outdoor therapy service, parents and referrers can be intrigued with our services for a number of reasons. There is a long history of taking at-risk youth to the outdoors for "character building" which we find problematic. For example, Kimball and Bacon (1993) thought it was the intentional use of stress that led wilderness therapy participants to a state of adaptation, thus helping them to become more adaptable to adversity. While this theory seems plausible, it leads parents, and practitioners accordingly, to focus on the stressing out of their therapy participants. To us, this hardly seems justifiable. Adding stress seems counterintuitive to the aims of good therapy (Mitten, 1994), which are about being in a better, calmer, and more stable place; better equipped to cope and find livable solutions. When a parent, or even a school, calls and states they want their young person to undergo a difficult and challenging experience to promote some sort of personal growth, we need to respond with understanding, while helping to guide the conversation back to the referrer's best hopes. Imagine thinking, "Could you do this work without intentionally stressing the young person? How would we know when we have done it?"

We have been asked by parents and schools for the similar *Brat Camp* (Russell, 2001) style programs some have seen on television. First off, most of those programs are accredited OBH programs and seem to have some perceived justifiable outcome research (DeMille et al., 2018). That said, we have to consider whether our outcomes can be accomplished without harming our young outdoor therapy participants. Our provision is not punitive in any way. Of course, therapy outcomes are achieved regularly, even under complex situations, without demoralizing or belittling the people we intend to help. Though parents may call with a particular narrative of what outdoor therapy looks like, we maintain our future focus. We continually ask what parents will notice if our services were indeed effective.

Additionally, we agree with Kurt Hahn's wise words (in Gookin, 2012) we shared at the start of this chapter. Sure, we could listen to a problem-saturated narrative and believe a certain young person *must* participate in our therapy. In some cases, the courts could say they must attend. We discuss with parents the importance of knowing what difference the therapy could make for their child and what they will notice if all goes well. We bring parents into the solution and work with the family to construct and notice experiences where the child feels needed and competent.

You can remind parents of the taxi metaphor presented by Bannink (2010). When we enter a taxi, our driver typically asks about our destination, not where we want to avoid, or how far away we want to go from where we are now. We want parents to describe the destination, not the problem. In the taxi, we do not want to say, "Take me anywhere but here. Just get me away." We want the address of where we are headed and a detailed understanding of how we will know when we arrive. We trust the taxi driver to take us there via the most efficient route.

Throughout the first consultation, we ask what parents will notice about their child, themselves, and the signs demonstrating that things are heading in the right direction. When animated, we ask parents, and the young person, how they were able to achieve these gains, though when addressing a possible future we stay clear of tasks, concentrating on the signs of moving in the preferred direction. Appendix K includes a short intake form we use to maintain the solution-focus while conducting an intake with parents and referrers. Like many working in clinical settings, we may be required to complete long-winded, objective assessments, and, rightfully, some sort of risk assessment, prior to taking a young person into therapy outdoors. You may find it useful to introduce these questions for maintaining a solution-focus from the initial conversation with parents.

"Homework" Assignments for Parents

We are not too fired up about the term *homework* in therapy. If a parent is not interested in the work you assign, they avoid it, just as young people might do. This can create a challenging transaction and lead you to wondering why a certain individual does not engage in your expert recommendation. Instead, we agree with Selekman (2005) in using the word *experiment*. When we return a client to their home from one of our adventures, parents may ask what happened during the session or what breakthrough occurred. Some will ask for tips on how you coped with all the bad behavior (Natynczuk, 2021). Why would we design a piece of work that did not offer opportunities for the client to be at their best, to experience a different way of being, and to gain glimpses of a path to a better future? Below are some ideas for responding to these specific requests.

The script below comes from True North Expeditions, Inc.'s *Parent Workbook*. The brief workbook allows parents to follow along during True North's 14-day expeditions (see Appendix L). Each day, parents are welcomed to complete a short solution-focused journal entry to help prepare for their adolescent's return. The aim of the activity is to utilize parents as key witnesses of change. We want them to explore what gives hope for future change and to notice it. We send this *Secret Detective* activity on day 13 of the 14-day program.

> "Your young person is returning home tomorrow. From our experience, they are most likely feeling excited, nervous, happy, sad, scared, and/or motivated. A lot of these feelings are probably occurring all at once.
>
> You have also made it through all of this information. We recommend keeping your responses for a gentle reminder from time to time. Remember, learning to walk is hard, and making changes is hard.
>
> So here is your final "Where to" assignment. Research has told us that parents see improvements when they set healthy and achievable boundaries (Note: With any teen, pick your battles wisely!). Adolescents want their efforts recognized and rewarded.
>
> This task is called the Sherlock Holmes' assignment. Now that your child is returning home, we need you to be our detective. We need you on red alert, looking for signs, no matter how big or small, indicating things are heading in the right direction.
>
> Write a list. The longer the better. When we return, we will touch base with you and talk about what you have found."

When parents complete these and similar tasks, we bring them in as expert witnesses of change and key allies.

A valuable opportunity to work with parents is gained by inviting them, with the young person's consent, to come along on the outdoor therapy session. I (Stephan) have observed what seem to be good-quality interactions between parent and child(ren) reported beyond the day of caving, climbing, or time in the woods. As much as possible, I ask the young person to direct the activity, especially when they can demonstrate some mastery of technique and local knowledge. Often, a location is chosen by the young person because they have experienced some particular success and want to demonstrate this expertise to parents. I find these sessions rewarding when I witness strengthening bonds and positive changes in the quality of relationships to include better communication and respect. Witnessing shared pleasure in the activity is always a bonus. Leadership is given over to the young person. They now host the event for as long as they want. We reflect on the experience afterwards. Parents and young participants can see and live through each other differently in this novel situation, one that generates exceptions, and opportunities to see and show their best selves.

Working in School Settings

Working with schools has been the mainstay of my (Stephan's) work since 1988. Mostly with one student and an adult helper, who might be a teaching assistant or an employee of my own. I have a Postgraduate Certificate in Education as a science teacher, which helps my work count as education provision within the broad heading of outdoor education. A typical session with a school is five to five and a half hours to fit in with the school day. All new students go through an induction day that also forms part of the risk assessment for each individual. We are lucky in the UK that so many types of adventure environments can be found without traveling too far. I use a large forest district, some 200 square miles in area, within a 45-minute drive from the school with cliffs, caves, iron mines, a river with interesting features, scrambles, lots of mature deciduous trees, and a variety of habitats for interesting temperate forest fauna. We work our way along a five-kilometer circuit over four hours, exploring as we go, and avoiding problem-focused talk. We chat about things that go well, what the participant enjoys doing, and the things they are good at. This induction gives an idea of the types of places we can go for off-road cycling, underground exploration, kayaking and canoeing, rock climbing, hill walking, bushcraft, and so on. The conversation is helpful to the building of a climate of confidence for this and subsequent sessions. Students gain a good idea of where we might go and what is involved in a day out adventuring. The induction day also gives me an idea of how much energy, stamina, curiosity, and safety awareness any given participant has, as well as insights into their social and emotional intelligence. Their *adventurosity* provides a rough index for the type and intensity of adventure activities I might suggest. After this induction day participants can choose from a menu of activities I am qualified and licensed to provide. There are bad weather options too, an indoor climbing wall or a variety of museums to visit.

Often the teaching assistant provided by the school benefits from the day too, especially if they assist long term. At the time of writing, my assistant, Chris, has overcome a significant fear of heights, and has developed technical skills I can rely on. Others have decided to qualify as teachers or change the direction of their career to work in outdoor education.

Ajmal and Ratner (2020) gave a useful review of working in a school environment with a solution-focused approach. We are interested in what happens when we invite young people out of school into the outdoors. We will assume there are safety protocols for off-site visits we must comply with, activity risk assessments, qualifications, licenses, and insurance. Call-out procedures are followed in case we are late returning, or might require a rescue. We also require appropriate local knowledge for the locations we use, such as where to park, where to get additional supplies, the nearest accident and emergency hospital, or best route through the narrow country lanes.

Based on our experience, it seems that there are two main types of referrals from schools. The first being a genuine request for a therapeutic intervention in which the young person is an active and consenting participant; the second being a way of getting a troublesome youth off-site for something that seems will be character forming, offering some traditional "alternative education" and giving the class a rest from one student's disruptive behavior. Young people of the latter category are often initially unaware about the therapeutic aspect of our work, though they do expect some fun from adventure and are generally happy to be out of school. They may hold some suspicion learning is involved.

It is far easier to have a therapeutic conversation with someone expecting it, less so with someone who likes the idea of the sessions, yet says they had no idea about the therapy. To increase hope and expectancy, we provide a rationale for how our therapy works and ensure co-adventurers understand we are interested in nothing other than being useful, no matter what that looks like (Frank & Frank, 1991). Working with a solution-focused mindset is, however, entirely possible as the language and tools we use in therapy are useful to coaching, mentoring, and teaching, and all add to the quality of the session, and work to build agency, hope, and social capital.

I have long been interested in the use of solution-focused tools in an un-spoken, experiential therapy, which can leave pupils feeling better in themselves, and with a useful increase in agency and self-efficacy though without difficult or "intrusive" conversations. Table 7.1 is developed from Natynczuk (2021) and gives examples of how solution-focused practice can be used through active involvement, to help participants experience themselves at their best and enjoy a "climate of competence."

Working with schools requires a careful attention to client experience, outcome, and the preferences of key stakeholders. Those who call you out to the school to adventure with one of their students are helpful as witnesses to change, as we describe below. Additionally, students may know they are in trouble, or a topic of concern, which is why you were summoned in the first place. To flip the script, make the first session meaningful, beyond the expectations of the student. Provide opportunities for moments we examined above. The following section will explore some solution-focused ideas for working across dynamic, multi-disciplinary teams.

Table 7.1 Examples of Outdoor Solution-Focused Concepts and Participant Experiences

Outdoor Solution-Focused Concepts	Participant Experiences
Exceptions – living exceptions to the challenges that brought the client to therapy	Participants can experience themselves as competent, curious, capable, and independent as skill and knowledge improve with experience outdoors.
Instances of preferred future and a lived glimpse of a different way of being: a path forward	Participants can experience themselves as calm, thoughtful, and helpful people, able to work through problems by negotiation and careful listening.
Demonstrating strengths, talents, "superpowers" that could be useful tools for change	Participants can experience being very good at something demanding skills and knowledge that is outside school, and with adults not dictating rules around how to be.
The practitioner becomes an active third person, able to give perspective on a client's own solutions	Sometimes questions about the future and what others would notice in the future are difficult for some participants to answer. Those events have not happened. For participants challenged by being asked to imagine events, it can be problematic to find a reliable third person perspective. This can be somewhat eased by ourselves providing a third person perspective with appropriate feedback from observations during the session. For example, "I saw how helpful you were with passing kit along that tight cave section, and how much your help was appreciated in getting us through the squeeze."

(Continued)

Table 7.1   Examples of Outdoor Solution-Focused Concepts and Participant Experiences (Cont'd)

Outdoor Solution-Focused Concepts	Participant Experiences
Suppose: coaching talk easily transposed into therapeutic talk	Questions, such as How do you know? Imagine you're coming down a section of rapids and you avoid that big rock. What would you see yourself doing? or How will you know today has been a good use of your time? are common for therapeutic conversations.
Living an authentic self with improved self-efficacy and agency as engagement improves	Confidence with taking responsibility, solving problems oneself, and giving leadership seem to help participants develop a durable sense of self-reliance.
Engaged for hours, or even days, at a time	This could be regarded as remarkable for participants known for an inability to concentrate and apply themselves in formal school lessons.
Reflection is in context and "natural mindfulness" (incidental, not timetabled) allows this	Mindfulness is reported to have many benefits, though can seem silly to some, whereas sitting quietly to observe deer, or salmon jumping, or cooking a sausage on a fire offer moments of mindfulness which come naturally.
Active and engaged co-adventurers sharing experiences in the moment	This is about instant and intrinsic reward, feeling good about successes in active learning and sharing it with others who appreciate the moment as it happens. Good engagement is key to the success of any therapy.

(Continued)

Table 7.1   Examples of Outdoor Solution-Focused Concepts and Participant Experiences (*Cont'd*)

Outdoor Solution-Focused Concepts	Participant Experiences
Not keeping problems alive and avoiding being solution-forced	We do not dwell on problems, or events that got the participant in trouble, only on strengths, resources, opportunities, and evidence of heading towards useful change.
Active collaboration and co-dependent journeying, taking responsibility for decisions and safety, trusting and respecting each other	Trust and respect are important components for the authentic co-dependency that begets further trust and respect. Here is part of the secret of forming a therapeutic alliance of quality.
Dignifying every participant's experience	We avoid teasing, joking, belittling people's efforts and gently and respectfully encourage all that goes well. Remember we are working therapeutically and not cajoling Olympian efforts.

Working with Other Helping Professionals

In 2015, I (Will) was contracted to provide consultation services for a high-profile case. The client, a 17-year-old named Bradley, was removed from his home at the age of two due to neglect and abuse. In fact, he was left in a dog kennel for most of his early childhood development and learning to crawl and walk were substantially delayed. After being removed to a foster home, his parents packed up and moved across state lines, preventing almost all further contact with their son. While becoming acquainted with this case, it is difficult to know what was worse: what happened before he was removed, or after.

By the time I met Bradley, he had attended 15 schools, endured more than ten breakdowns in foster care, was arrested on multiple occasions for destruction of property and substance use, and was moved from one residential facility to the next. The lack of progress in his care led to a state government inquiry into the most difficult child protection cases over the previous 20 years. Bradley was one of four case studies utilized.

Bradley's clinical psychologist, who had worked with him since his childhood, called me. She heard of my work with adolescents and provided an in-depth conceptualization of the case, as well as hundreds of pages of notes and assessment, ranging from his trauma to learning difficulties to cognitive delays. This is probably born out of my own arrogance, or ignorance, but I felt honored to be invited to help. "Let us do something different," I thought.

I sat with Bradley in a decrepit agency in one of the rougher parts of town. My bulldog was with me who he liked and behaved with appropriately. I asked about his best hopes for our work together. "I want an adventure," he said. "None of my carers let me adventure, or they don't know what they're doing." I thought that was awesome. We were already a good fit! I asked where he wanted to go, and he told me of a place in the bush he would hike to with the best youth worker he ever had. Our initial consultation ended, and I drove home.

Along the way, the psychologist called to ask how things went. "Really well! We're going on a hike next week," I replied.

"I was fearing this." She was mortified. "He will be triggered and retraumatized sitting in the car with you. It is like the kennel where he experienced the abuse." This made sense to me. After all, I am well versed in the treatment of complex trauma and Australia's guidelines for such treatment (Kezelman & Stavropoulos, 2012). I thought I better listen to her. She had known Bradley for years.

The following morning, I woke up to a call from the receptionist where I met Bradley the day before. "He is here for your hike, Will," she said. "When can I expect you?" Bradley did not understand which day we would meet, so over the telephone, I began having the receptionist schedule the meeting on Bradley's phone for the following week. Bradley told me he had printed the Google map of where we were going. This struck me as an opportunity.

"Screw it," I thought. Tomorrow was a day set aside for supervision, consultation with outdoor therapy providers, and writing.

"Bradley, nevermind. Come back tomorrow. I'll move some stuff around and see you then."

He showed up on time. Bradley was ready to go. He brought a water bottle, sunscreen, and even a Swiss Army knife. Most of the people I work with were never this prepared. We had a great time. His carers called to let me know they had not seen him so happy. Instead of staying up all night playing video games, he went to sleep at 9:30pm. We continued working together for months. He was engaging with the community mental health organization's education program and proceeding with his studies. Everyone was happy. Tragically, Bradley's past caught up to him and he was associated with an event of gang violence from the year before. Cameras proved it.

"I've changed!" he pleaded to the judge in the courtroom where we all advocated for what we had noticed. Bradley was locked away. As a repeat offender, the sentence was more strict, and our work together was over. After the devastating news, the treatment team, including the original psychologist, went to a local cafe to figure out what happened. "I told you this would not work," she said. She anticipated failure all along. We lost contact with one another, despite such a promising, though annihilating, experience.

As I reflected on Bradley's case and experience in government care, I grew angry and frustrated. All the assessments, expensive services, and government inquiries resulted in a story of trauma and pain. Why was someone who was involved in this case for more than ten years still leading the way, despite no progress? Should I have engaged in the piles of problem-focused assessments the way I had? After all, what conceptualization of Bradley's history was useful towards outcomes? Virtually none. How could a solution-focus have helped me to put all of this into perspective? Within this story, there are many implications for our work, and interdisciplinary approaches to helping. In this section, we will examine our approach to working with problem-focused practitioners and how we can position a referrer as a *second client*.

Working with Problem-Focused Practitioners

Informed by the work of Berg and Steiner (2003), Bannink (2010) provided implications for working with practitioners who may not be familiar with solution-focused approaches. We have found it useful to implement these concepts in our work as many of our co-adventurers are referred to us after many treatment failures. Like Bradley, many will come with *Fat File Syndrome*, large case records with numerous diagnosed mental disorders, lists of symptomatic behaviors, and descriptions of dysfunctional family systems. The practitioner on the other end of the phone may feel frustrated or a sense of shame based on their client's lack of change. Always begin by empathizing with the efforts of the practitioner. After all, most practitioners struggle to fail successfully, a way of getting the client to a more engaging, helpful service or worker. We discuss this further in Chapter 9. Below are some ideas for facilitating discussions with such practitioners.

- Stay focused on your client's best hopes and preferences. This is the map and compass used to avoid getting lost in the woods. It is tempting and easy to fall into a diagnostic trap, engaging in lengthy discussions about how resistant, unmotivated, or traumatized the client is. Set a goal for the discussion, ask solution-focused questions, and adopt a future focus. When we hear the practitioner's best hopes, we ask them to notice when small changes occur.
- Provide compliments to the other practitioners. Focus on collaboration and try to notice the progress that was made. For example, if the client continues to attend a counselor's session despite the lack of progress, it is wonderful the practitioner is seeking your support to help their client.
- Ask about what has worked in the past. When was their client most engaged in their work together? What was noticed when most progress was made?
- Throughout the meeting, we like to provide appreciative summaries, as described in Chapter 5. Demonstrate to practitioners you are listening and point out what is working and everyone's best hopes for your involvement in the case. Avoid *why* or closed-ended questions as these can be interpreted as judgmental.

Andy was a 25-year-old who had grown up in foster care. He was diagnosed with fetal alcohol spectrum disorder and resided in a supportive living home. The psychiatrist overseeing his case called for the possibility of a short group expedition for Andy to interact with others his own age. He was high functioning but tended to isolate and had low self-esteem. Instead of focusing on the problem narrative, we asked the psychiatrist his best hopes for Andy's participation on the program. He hoped Andy would feel more confident, which would be evidenced by possibly joining a sporting club or simply leaving the home more often. After the expedition, we sent the psychiatrist an email asking him to pay attention to the times when Andy exhibited this improved confidence. The psychiatrist called and said he loved the rock climbing portion of the expedition and asked for his support worker to take Andy to the indoor climbing gym. Andy asked his flat-mate to go with him on his next visit and they learned about a weekend climbing program for people with disabilities. Andy's social network grew.

Referrers as a Second Client

Just like the example with Andy's psychiatrist, we are used to working with doctors, disability support workers, psychotherapists, schoolteachers, principals, probation officers, and parents. Similar to the problem-focused practitioner, referrers may have pre-determined ideas and preconceived outcomes for their client engaging in our service. When working with "involuntary" clients, such as in substance use services, it is common for a referrer's ideas to dominate the case conceptualization. The probation officer may ensure the adolescent's attendance on a court-mandated expedition. The school may threaten to expel the student if they do not engage in therapy and improve their attendance. While we remain focused on the best hopes of our co-adventurers, we know that success or failure will likely be determined, maybe incorrectly so, by the referrer. You can use the Referral Worksheet in Appendix K as a template for speaking with referrers. This can help you to stay focused.

Chevalier (1995) described referrers as a second client. We should collaborate with them, seek their advice, and build a cooperative relationship. Ask if the referrer is willing to work together towards the best outcome for the client. We inquire about when the client's problem that spurred the referral was absent or reduced. We want to hear about anything except when the problem is worse. Position the referrer as a partner and witness of change. Remember, these additional "clients" make up the web of interested parties we can discuss in supervision (see Chapter 10).

Relationships do not only matter with co-adventurers, but also with the helping professionals in your community. To grow a thriving practice, relationships are everything. We avoid the falsehood that what we do is more special than any other clinician. As described throughout this book, there is probably little evidence to support such a stance. Like the turf battles occurring between the nearly 1,000 different models of therapy, this stance is unlikely to build bridges in your professional network. When working in a school, we focus our attention on how hard teachers are working to keep students engaged, some with budgets akin to the smell of an oily rag. We keep complaints about curriculum and the unjust pressures placed on young people to ourselves, or a friendly discussion in teachers' breakout rooms. Collaborating with external helping professionals is about finding common ground. If we over-inflate our own self-assessment, we are unlikely to gain the professional and clinical humility to hand stuck cases back to those who have referred to us previously.

Conclusion

It can be tempting to perceive what we do with a co-adventurer in isolation to those in their lives. Third party narratives and key witnesses to change are resources the solution-focused practitioner can take advantage of. They are invested in the change process but may be demoralized due to a lack of hope that our services can help. The more we can do to increase the expectancy for change, the better. In this chapter, we provided techniques and considerations for engaging with parents and referrers. Where our practice has mostly centered on working with adolescents, we spend a lot of our time using our solution-focus to engage those supporting the young person's development.

From here, we move on from focusing on specific contexts or treatment settings to provide ideas for how we conceptualize and improve our effectiveness. The following chapter examines the core competencies for outdoor therapy practice and provides some strategies for avoiding burnout.

References

Ajmal, Y., & Ratner, H. (2020). *Solution focused practice in schools: 80 ideas and strategies*. Routledge.

Bacon S. B., & Kimball R. (1989). The wilderness challenge model. In R. D. Lyman, S. Prentice-Dunn, & S. Gabel (Eds.), *Residential and inpatient treatment of children and adolescents* (pp. 115–144). Springer. https://doi.org/10.1007/978-1-4899-0927-5_7

Bannink, F. (2010). *1001 solution-focused questions: Handbook for solution-focused interviewing*. W. W. Norton & Co.

Berg, I. K., & Steiner, T. (2003). *Children's solution work*. W. W. Norton & Co.

Chevalier, A. J. (1995). *On the client's path: A manual for the practice of solution-focused therapy*. New Harbinger Publications, Inc.

DeMille, S., Tucker, A. R., Gass, M. A., Javorski, S., VanKanegan, C., Talbot, B., & Karoff, M. (2018). The effectiveness of outdoor behavioral healthcare with struggling adolescents: A comparison group study. A contribution for the special issue: "Social innovation in child and youth services". *Children and Youth Services Review, 88*, 241–248. https://doi.org/10.1016/j.childyouth.2018.03.015

Frank, J. D., & Frank, J. B. (1991). *Persuasion and healing: A comparative study of psychotherapy*. JHU Press.

Gass, M. A., Gillis, H. L., & Russell, K. C. (2012). *Adventure therapy: Theory, research, and practice*. Routledge.

Gookin, J. (2012). *NOLS wilderness wisdom* (2nd ed.) Stackpole Books.

Kezelman, C., & Stavropoulos, P. (2012). *Practice guidelines for treatment of complex trauma and trauma informed care and service delivery*. Adults Surviving Child Abuse.

Mitten, D. (1994). Ethical considerations in adventure therapy: A feminist critique. *Women & Therapy, 15*(3–4), 55–84. https://doi.org/10.1300/J015v15n03_06

Natynczuk, S. (2021). Co-adventuring for change: A solution-focused framework for "unspoken" therapy outdoors. *Relational Child and Youth Care Practice, 34*(4), 58–66.

Russell, K. C. (2001). What is wilderness therapy? *Journal of Experiential Education, 24*, 70–79. https://doi.org/10.1177%2F105382590102400203

Selekman, M. D. (2005). *Pathways to change: Brief therapy with difficult adolescents* (2nd ed.). Guilford Publishing.

Part III

From Good Enough to Excellence

8

Core Competencies and Professionalism

"The difference between something good and something great is attention to detail."

Charles Swindoll (2000, p. 305)

How practitioners construct their professional identity around their competences has long been an interest of mine (Stephan). When I researched adventure therapy practitioners' perceptions of professionalism (Natynczuk, 2016, 2020) I was struck by, and heartened, to learn how convergent the evolution of professional practice was in our multi-discipline, diverse, and eclectic specialty. All that with so little formal multi-disciplinary, or cross-disciplinary training, or specific qualification or accreditation for outdoor therapy providers.

In 2013, I decided to up my business skills and signed up for a part-time Executive Master of Business Administration (MBA) at a local university. I had been running my practice without really understanding what I was doing in terms of business theory at any depth for far too long.

Everything was trial and error. Some ideas worked and paid off, others did not. This wasted energy, time, money, and no doubt opportunities. The MBA opened my eyes to business theory, good practice, and tools to drive innovation. Three years later, I wrote my dissertation examining how adventure-based practitioners perceived professionalism and how they built it for themselves. Practitioners were invited to self-identify as professionals in adventure, bush, outdoor, or wilderness therapy to describe how they assembled their qualifications, accreditations, ethics, and memberships to governing bodies, and so on. They described how they maintained professional standards and personal development.

DOI: 10.4324/9781003217558-11

Perhaps we will eventually see balanced, cross-disciplinary, robust accrediting bodies for therapy outdoors in each nation, or maybe regional collections of countries with similar outlooks and practice models, such as what is occurring with the Nordic countries. There is no certainty this will happen though as at the time of writing, there are so few of us for the critical mass needed to fund and administer a dedicated organization. Until then, practitioners must hold separate awards for adventure leadership and their therapeutic modality. In the United Kingdom, it is common for National Governing Body (NGB) membership for adventure leaders, guides, coaches, and instructors to come with guidelines on professional behavior, codes of conduct, and something about ethics. However, in the UK, NGBs for adventure sports are generally awarding bodies, not professional membership organizations. Some practitioners do belong to professional governing bodies for therapy, each with their own disciplinary procedures in the case of unsafe practice. In contrast, some adventure sport qualifications can be held without being a member of a governing body. In other circumstances, competence may be enough if demonstrated and vouched for otherwise. Ultimately, practitioners are answerable to government and health policies in their respective cultural context.

Legislation varies from nation to nation. Some nations are more rigorous with policing adventure qualifications than counseling and therapy regulations, others vice versa. The Association for Experiential Education (AEE) Certified Clinical Adventure Therapist (CCAT) Credential Certification (2021) is slowly gathering momentum in the USA though with limited international reach, certainly where established accreditation has more authority and carries more weight. The UK's Institute for Outdoor Learning (IOL) has similarly attempted to codify Outdoor Mental Health Interventions (Richards et al., 2020). Neither AEE nor IOL are governing bodies for therapy, though they are well respected for their influence and advocacy for outdoor learning.

The IOL advises that:

> its members will provide honest and transparent information about how both psychotherapy and outdoor elements of practice are resourced and delivered. They would need to demonstrate and publish public information on the type of approach, and related qualifications and competencies as appropriate to communicate this. This is not designed to discourage practices across the different zones of the model, but what it does mean is participants are accurately informed of the type of practice on offer and can make informed decisions in terms of participation and manage expectations accordingly.
>
> (Richards et al., 2020, p. 6)

The IOL has produced worthy guidelines though, as they point out, practitioners must rely on their qualifications from established institutions. In the UK, we have a robust licensing system for providers of outdoor adventure, which came about in response to a large number of deaths from an instructed kayaking accident in Lyme Bay (Bennett, 1993).Water sports instructors, guides, and coaches must demonstrate competence in their chosen discipline by gaining, firstly, skills awards, then instructor and coaching awards. This is similar for mountain, rock climbing, off-road cycling, and caving awards in the UK where skills assessments form part of the leadership qualification: the uppermost awards demanding a very high, even exceptional, degree of skills, ability, experience, and knowledge. This introduces a further complication over terminology whereby in some countries one can use the term "guide" for someone who leads with little knowledge, ability, and experience. In some European countries in hiring a guide one would expect an exceptionally qualified mountaineer, caver, climber, canoeist, or rafter. Becoming a guide in the UK, France, and Italy is not easy, training for assessment is often a full-time occupation, and requires living in the mountains for at least a year to prepare for the assessment. The IOL guidelines are correct to point out that practitioners have to be nothing less than transparent about their capabilities to safely lead adventures in remote places, and their qualifications and experience to deliver helpful therapy at the same time.

National Governing Bodies for counseling and psychotherapy are, by comparison, much more rigorous with their codes of conduct and policies on ethics, such that membership or accreditation can be withdrawn for bad practice and other misdemeanors amounting to gross misconduct (Caldwell, 2015). Requirements for accountability in particular differentiate a professional body from an awarding body for adventure activities. Having said that, the highest awards are often held by people working professionally with adventure in the outdoors. Uniting these two overlapping circles of counseling and adventure in a Venn diagram for a single NGB for outdoor therapy is a fundamental step in professionalizing our adventure therapy specialty. That said, finding consensus in an ever-diversifying international field makes this less than likely. Until then it is important to be independently qualified and accredited as a professional in whatever modality suits you best, as without that, practitioners are not accountable for bad practice in their therapeutic work.

In Part III of this book, we use our research and experience to examine the ideals of the "good enough" practitioner to one that strives for excellence. We begin here with a presentation about the keys to proficiency and discuss core competencies. This has emerged from research and our experiences working in various cultural contexts. These, like all things in outdoor therapy, are up for debate. We do not propose a rigid framework all practitioners must adopt. We recommend practitioners reflect on these competencies in relation to their own practice, experience, and knowledge. As we go on to discuss burnout and what practitioners can do to avoid such dire circumstances, we build some frameworks for striving to improve our work and becoming better outdoor practitioners.

12 Keys of Proficiency

The keys are briefly summarized in Table 8.1. As you read these, you can use Appendix M in the field manual to examine which areas of your practice are worthy of further development.

We do not propose to talk in depth about all of the 12 Keys in this book, just to flag those key components while we concentrate on co-adventuring for change. Practitioners should pay regard to the 12 Keys as wider aspects of competence to add depth in terms of both theoretical and practical frameworks.

Knowledge of philosophy brings additional meaning to one's work and can help co-adventurers construct meaning for their adventure, nature-based, wilderness, and outdoor therapy. Pedagogy helps one understand the education and learning aspects of your work. Paying attention to how people learn and how we teach basic outdoor skills can help maintain a good therapeutic alliance by avoiding being inappropriately didactic and authoritarian. Ethics are essential to good practice and without an ethical code, and real consequences for breaking it, there is no hope for becoming a member of a professional body. Do not treat ethics as an unfortunate or burdensome reality. One can be professional in one's practice in terms of values and quality of practice, yet not belong to a profession, though we ask where people complain about bad therapy and get reparations for dangerous practices. Managing risk relates to both psychological and physical risk of harm. Risk management practices may influence insurance premiums and coverage. Regulating authorities may inspect policies, safety procedures, staff qualifications, and training before issuing a license to work remotely with vulnerable populations.

Counseling skills are obviously a requirement and research shows all modalities are similarly effective. What matters is the skill of the practitioner and

Table 8.1 12 Keys of Proficiency in Outdoor Therapy

12 Keys	Meaning
Philosophy	Practitioners need a general guiding orientation for finding meaning in their work, perhaps drawing on social construction and existentialism, for example. Read widely to explore other thinkers' experiences and how those influenced their search for meaning in life. There is such a rich literature on philosophy going back thousands of years. One might start with Socratic questioning, entertain Stoicism, and so on. We recommend reading something that may challenge you, not just what you already align with.
Pedagogy	Knowledge of how we share and receive information, how social constructs help and hinder learning, and how learning can be layered on what is already understood are important to how "education" occurs as an enjoyable, useful experience. The classic schools of Social Constructivism, Behaviorism, and Liberation Pedagogy are useful ideas to explore and to help understand practitioner-client relationships, especially when it comes to teaching outdoor skills. Additionally, if you align with experiential learning, as many do, focus on how this mode of learning and teaching relates to therapy experiences.
Ethics	Ethics are the values and qualities that guide our behavior, especially in respect to fairness, discrimination, privilege, equanimity, and so on. Practitioners should align to the codes of ethics presented in their professional association. Your job description is one way to focus your ethics. However, practitioners should reflect on their professional values in relation to what their bosses ask them to do. Is it possible you are being asked to practice in certain unethical ways? Practicing at odds to your ethical values is an easy road to burnout.

(Continued)

Table 8.1   12 Keys of Proficiency in Outdoor Therapy (*Cont'd*)

12 Keys	*Meaning*
Managing Risk and Insurance	Be mindful of what brings harm to you, your clients, and third persons, emotionally, psychologically, and physically, and mitigating the risk of damage being done. Robust risk assessments and safety protocols are developed to record one's thinking and reduce the chances of harm. Safety procedures further document how practitioners go about staying safe, including replacement of equipment, qualifications needed to run certain activities, levels of supervision, and so on. Some insurance companies will ask for risk assessments and might refuse to insure against risks or increase premiums accordingly. Insurance companies effectively control what is possible for therapy outdoors. It is essential to match risks with insurance coverage and to reflect on the consequences of harm to people and property, or loss of equipment. Do not avoid the minutiae of your operation to ensure your insurance coverage is adequate. Have in mind the cost of repatriation and emergency evacuation. When overlooked, this has proven to be very expensive.
Counseling Skills	We have written about the many varieties of counseling skills available. Deliberately work towards becoming proficient at whatever modality you favor, use feedback-informed treatment, and most importantly remember to be human first, and therapist second. Schedule time throughout each week to practice and develop your skills deliberately. Clinical practice is not 'deliberate practice.'
Therapeutic Alliance	Everything a practitioner does impacts the quality of the working relationship between client and practitioner. One has to be careful to maintain a good alliance as this is a good predictor of outcomes. Taking therapy outdoors can be good for building trust, mutual reliance, and respect. It is easy to damage the alliance with misplaced leadership, or inadequate technical expertise. Ask your client if they are getting what they need from your work. If they are not finding your work helpful, do something different, or refer them onwards.

(Continued)

Table 8.1   12 Keys of Proficiency in Outdoor Therapy (*Cont'd*)

12 Keys	*Meaning*
Technical Competence	From knot tying to navigation in limited visibility, surfing a wave in a canoe to fire lighting by friction, technical skills have to be practiced and perfected, especially those needed for rescue. Gaining qualifications is typically the requisite that employers of instructors, adventure sport coaches, and leaders seek, more so than a degree in adventure leadership. There are occasions when teaching technical skills can be therapeutic, such when some mastery is gained, or when life-saving skills are learned.
Adventure Leadership	There is a fine balance between adventure leadership and working therapeutically. Lead badly and there could be dire consequences. Perhaps someone gets hurt. Do bad therapy, and someone leaves your session in a worse condition than when they arrived. The balance is about protecting the therapeutic alliance, so leadership should be enabling and liberating, just like your therapeutic practice.
Continuing Professional Development	One has to stay on top of recent developments relating to therapeutic practice and outdoor facilitation. This includes continuing to have your own adventures as much as it does pursuing higher leadership awards and attending such events as the International Adventure Therapy Conference. In addition, carve out time to attend events from diverging theoretical frameworks to challenge your professional growth.
Supervision	Finding a good supervisor is essential. Finding someone accredited in counseling supervision to a master's standard who understands the context of your work is priceless. A good supervisor will take in all aspects of your work, including stakeholders and those who influence your practice. Having professional scrutiny of your work keeps you sharp, makes sure your work is ethical, boundaried, current, well-informed, and safe for you and your clients.

(Continued)

Table 8.1   12 Keys of Proficiency in Outdoor Therapy (*Cont'd*)

12 Keys	*Meaning*
Business Administration	This category extends far beyond being efficient with paperwork. Understanding marketing will pay huge dividends for your business effectiveness. This includes knowing your purpose, understanding who your clients are and are not, where to find them, aligning your values with your measurable mission statement, auditing what works and doing more of it, networking, publishing, and speaking where it makes a difference, and performing regular assessments of your commercial viability. The list is long, and it may be worth enrolling on a business studies course.
Self-Care and Avoiding Burnout	If you are not looking after yourself, it is going to be challenging to look out for others. Take self-care seriously and plan days for rest, regeneration, and improvement. Having your own adventures (without clients) has to be mandatory. Attend to your "fulfillment of purpose" and nurture it relentlessly.

how much effort the practitioner puts into staying on top of their game. That includes asking clients if the therapy was any good for them and doing something about putting it right. This neatly brings us to the quality of the therapeutic alliance, including how well clients are engaged and participating in the therapy, no matter the type. How much technical competence is required depends on the safety needed to be in place, so no one gets hurt during an adventure. To be fluent, practitioners may need to learn about knots, search and rescue, adventure-specific rescue techniques, first aid, navigation, and so on. Credentials vouch for one's competence.

Adventure leadership is a subject with many iterations. Host leadership is an appropriate model for our work with solution-focused practice at its foundation and a helpful opportunity to align our therapeutic modality with a leadership model (Natynczuk, 2019).

Staying up to speed with current developments is essential. This goes not just for developments in the therapy of our choice and informing your practice based on the best available evidence, but equally applies to adventure skills. We cannot stress enough the importance of having your own adventures. As self-employed practitioners, we have found it difficult at times to say no to work, or worse, to take part in our own adventures without feeling guilty for time away from work and family. This situation lasted for me (Stephan) about two decades. An inspector of my adventure activities license told me I needed to demonstrate my continued efforts to train at a level above the one I mostly operated at in my day-to-day work. This was the permission I needed to have my own adventures in the guise of continuing professional practice. I felt such relief. I needed to hear it from another professional.

The 12 Keys are a framework for development. We recommend using the field manual and planning areas to further your evolution as an outdoor therapy practitioner. While it may seem counterintuitive, your professional development is a key to avoid automaticity and burnout. The danger in being simply "competent" is that in challenging situations, we will revert to whatever it is we do automatically. We need to push ourselves to the edge of our performance and learning (Miller et al., 2020). In the section that follows, we will examine how striving for excellence is one of the best antidotes to burnout.

Burnout and Avoiding Burnout

Burnout is of special interest to us. It begins insidiously, slowly creeping up, and barely noticed like a crocodile until too late, snap! It has you in its jaws and it is difficult to break free. Burnout begins with a noticeable decline in interest in your work, increasing loss of motivation, and increasing disengagement. As disinterest changes to difficulty, absenteeism becomes an attractive option. At this point your employment is at risk. Next, missing a couple of paychecks and your accommodation is at risk. Depression can follow with the accompanying loss of hope, and personal relationships might be at risk too. Burnout is serious and should not be ignored as an existential threat.

We have witnessed how bad this can be, especially when it reaches the stage of almost total disengagement from others and loss of motivation for even mundane tasks. Obviously, this is dangerous for the individual. It is also an avoidable loss of knowledge, skills, experience, and expertise for the field as practitioners might well seek employment doing something completely different.

Schwenk and Natynczuk (2015) described a number of factors contributing to burnout. The same prime factors pertaining to indoor therapy apply outdoors. Combining published factors and our observations, these are some of the indicators to look for:

- Sense of ineffectiveness and that work is pointless, diminution of purpose.
- Lack of alignment in values and aims, also between practitioner and employer.
- Few resources and an absence of support from management to fulfill work.
- Vague strategic planning or poor execution of planning from the employer.
- Poor contracting, such that it feels impossible to meet expectations.
- Poor relationships with colleagues.
- A feeling of being undervalued and that efforts are unappreciated.
- Inability to fulfill any sense of purpose.

Effective clinical supervision focused on your professional development and self-care can help slow, even reverse burnout before personal counseling and perhaps medication become indicated. This is only part of the remedy and will not be enough to tackle institutional failings, such as poor strategic execution of business strategy. There is an energy that comes from a collective sense of purpose and appreciation of supportive teamwork. Fortunately, solution-focused practice lends itself to business coaching. Kirsten Dierolf and Mark McKergow, among others, are internationally recognized for their work as business coaches and demonstrate the versatility of solution-focused practice to bring about change. The lesson seems to be that a theoretically aligned systemic approach is wise.

For those in private practice, burnout manifests itself through a decline in diligence around administrative tasks: not opening letters, taking too long to answer emails and enquiries, sensing a lack of energy and enthusiasm, and over-sleeping. We cannot emphasize enough the importance of self-care. In our own experience, it can be difficult to grant oneself permission for adventures. It helped to be told that our own adventures were part of our continuing professional development. Of course, we knew this, though we still needed to hear this from another professional. Second to this is the challenge of choosing with whom we adventure for our own self-care as it can feel like work if all the technical and safety decisions fall on us, the outdoor professional.

How One Gets Their Groove Back

It is a special occasion. Maybe your birthday or anniversary or you have graduated from university. To celebrate, you and a special someone decide the time is right to go try that restaurant in town everyone is talking about. You have heard about their new spring menu with fresh produce coming from their organic farm only a few miles from where you live. As you enter through a heavy dark door, you are greeted with a smile and an offer to store your coat. It was raining outside and no one else was wearing Gore-Tex indoors.

You take notice of the attention to detail. Every glass is polished to perfection. The flowers on your table are as fresh as possible and the linen napkins pressed and folded impeccably. As each meal arrives, you notice the precision in which the chef and their team have plated each item, from the julienned heirloom carrot to the clarity of the tomato consommé, which is served with a vegetable cannelloni.

You feel special, and rightfully so. You are there to celebrate. Despite your order, there are special treats brought to your table. A sneaky glass of bubbles to welcome you, and a few dark chocolate covered coffee beans to end the meal, despite feeling too full to order dessert.

Yes, here is another food metaphor, probably linking seamlessly to host leadership (McKergow & Pugliese, 2019). Maintaining a Michelin star rating as a top restaurant in the world is hard, really hard. It takes a leader who pushes their team to strive for excellence. There can be no off night. These restaurants are consistently judged and observed. They must work impossibly hard to obtain one star, let alone maintain their rating or improve.

People join the helping professions to make a difference. Early on in their career they note a keen ability to build meaningful relationships and help people achieve their preferred future. If they did not, they would have a hard time waking up every morning and getting themselves to work. Here lies a problem. Most people, regardless of their training, are effective practitioners at an average level (Miller et al., 2020). Again, psychotherapy outcomes on average are good, yet no one wants to be an average therapist. The problem is that it is hard to get better. Consider Olympians who spend years shaving milliseconds off their racing results from the four years prior. Their efforts are honed on becoming just a tiny bit faster.

Heather was a social worker employed at a large non-profit organization in rural Australia. She managed a small team of practitioners working primarily with Indigenous youth. She contracted me (Will) for consultation as she felt the service needed some fresh energy. She butt heads with her line manager who told her the agency needed to be world class and would not acknowledge the problems impacting day-to-day service delivery.

After a brief consultation with Stephan, I held a meeting with Heather, the manager, and the team of practitioners. I asked future focused questions about their best hopes and what they will notice to indicate the consultation was worthwhile. The practitioners all described being able to simply do their work, instead of focusing on key performance indicators meaningless to their co-adventurers. Heather mentioned risk management practices becoming more streamlined as the line manager was quite risk averse, and getting permission to work outdoors with this population, which they preferred, was met with resistance from the manager. They were all working in ways that did not align with how they felt at their best.

"I mean I am not an outdoorsy person," the line manager acknowledged. She went on to describe what her pursuit of building a world-leading service meant. It was difficult to follow. I asked how everyone would define world leading and what they would notice if they were to reach such a standard. Heather spoke about engagement, one practitioner argued for safe and impactful outdoor therapy practice. After some discussion, we agreed on one thing. To ever reach world leading, we have to know where we are now. We needed a baseline.

For a few months I helped the agency begin to evaluate their services using outcome monitoring. Whenever a certain case was at risk, judging by the client feedback, we met to develop a plan to either adapt our work or help the young person find a more appropriate service. It was a humbling process for some. Based on the feedback, the outdoor therapy clients seemed to really enjoy their time outdoors and maintained strong relational bonds with the staff. However, when they were asked how important and meaningful the work was therapeutically, the data dropped off.

We revisited our mission statement of being world leading and held a frank and open discussion focused on the fact our data showed we had a way to go. I asked who was ready to work diligently to get better. Everyone agreed. Within two weeks, however, the line manager resigned, and Heather was promoted to the position. The agency continued eliciting client feedback and strived to be world leading. They now have better staff retention than many programs I know and in 2019, they secured five years' worth of government funding and an award for youth justice programs. Heather was given more money to play with.

When I sit with Heather and talk about her work, she always brings up how important it was to stop talking about being the best and build the data to get better. Being the best is a process, not a destination. When she knows the areas in need of improvement, she is able to ask for help from her friends and colleagues and develop plans of action. She realized that it was the status quo that was hurting her passion, not the young people or her team. Heather wanted to be the best and knew deep down that she and her team were not. It was brave to measure what mattered most, the co-adventurers' perception of relationship and outcome, and to use the data to get better.

Staying on top of your game is important. This involves a usual cast of characters, such as good supervision or coaching, focusing on client experiences, going the extra mile for someone, and informing your practice with the best available evidence. Next, we build data about our own effectiveness. Not the effectiveness of outdoor therapy as a whole, your effectiveness. The following chapter examines a ready-to-implement method for doing this.

Now we have presented a "strengths-based" framework throughout this book, but we are going to turn this on its head when it comes to burnout and professional development. Building evidence can be scary. "Am I as effective as I think?" "What if a client says something that hurts my feelings?" We have two responses. First, if you find out you are eliciting average outcomes or that you have some clear areas requiring improvement, great! We can develop a plan to build on these areas and you will reap the benefits. Your co-adventurers are better off for it as you begin challenging yourself at your learning and performing edge to improve your effectiveness.

Second, if what a client shares challenges you, great! This indicates you have contributed to building a relationship and climate in your work that the person feels supported enough to tell you the truth. Congratulations! On a serious note, practitioners should want to know if people are disengaged or feeling that their work is off track. Upon building your data relating to your outdoor therapy practice, we highly recommend developing plans to get better.

Mathieu et al. (2015) argued that to avoid burnout, we must know who on our caseload is disengaged. Continuing to work with someone who is not benefitting from our work is not only at odds with our professional ethics, it is a recipe for disaster. We will discuss how we remain open to finding a more appropriate practitioner when stuck, rather than crossing our fingers and hoping something will stick. Remember, the longer we work with someone who is not benefitting, the less likely any change will occur.

So, what can we learn from the Michelin star restaurants? Remember, we are hosting people's outdoor experiences. Outdoor therapy practitioners make decisions about equipment, food, and risk management strategies. These contribute to the experiences of the co-adventurers. Like Swindoll's (2000) quote beginning this chapter, striving for excellence and maintaining a precise attention to detail, both in the empirical outcomes you elicit and the feedback you receive from co-adventurers helps you stay on the top of your game and keep you engaged. If you slip back into automatic practice, day in and day out, the rat race if you will, burnout creeps in.

Burnout is not necessarily the result of being busy, or overworked, though it can be. More often than not, it is the result of working at odds to our own practice values (Mathieu et al., 2015). When we have disengaged people on our caseload, we dread their presence. The value that brought us to this work is about helping people and believing in their best selves. To continue working with them may not only invite a poor outcome, it makes us fear going to work.

Many people take their work outdoors because of their relationship and kinship with nature. They want to share their passion and love for outdoor environments and adventures with others in some kind of remediating way. When things go wrong or we work in ways that challenge our professional values, we see practitioners leave the field. Or worse, they stay and hate their work. Their love for the outdoors is diminished by missing out on some of the early warning signs. As burnout finds its way into our daily lives, our attention to detail declines.

Conclusion: A Note on Professionalism in Outdoor Therapy

It is important to make a note here about privilege. The idea of learning from Michelin starred restaurants as a metaphor for outdoor therapy practices assumes that any of us have been to such an establishment or had the opportunity to afford such an experience. Moreover, many therapeutic practitioners work for under-funded agencies where allocated funding is used to simply cover the bones of the business, let alone supplementing initiatives to improve client engagement. We also acknowledge that Michelin starred chefs tend to be white men (Lee, 2019). We are not only intrigued by the metaphors from Eurocentric, fine dining experiences, we are intrigued by any endeavor striving for excellence in their respective field.

The metaphor here is about holding ourselves to the highest standards, despite funding restraints. Said another way, clients in private practice tend to have one session a week. Practitioners working full time may have up to eight sessions a day. That could be 30 sessions a week! Time allocated to writing up our notes, returning a phone call, supervision, or opening the mail becomes limited. Co-adventurers may be excited for their one experience with you each week. They are unaware of how busy you have been and all the work that took place behind the scenes. We imagine each encounter with a client, most importantly at session one but also at session 30, as an opportunity to increase our attention to detail and focus on their experience. It is their adventure, not ours.

In this chapter, we presented the 12 Keys to proficiency and encouraged practitioners to use the field manual to develop plans for continued professional development. We reconsidered burnout and the importance of holding ourselves to the highest standard. We have set the stage for the importance of embracing our role as evidence builders and present a user-friendly framework for building said data in the following chapter.

References

Bennett, W. (1993, March 24). The school canoe tragedy: Canoe instructors were not qualified teachers: No official checks on centres offering activity holidays. *The Independent*. Retrieved from www.independent.co.uk/news/uk/the-school-canoe-tragedy-canoe-instructors-were-not-qualified-teachers-no-official-checks-on-centres-offering-activity-holidays-1499567.html

Caldwell, B. E. (2015). *Saving psychotherapy: How therapists can bring the talking cure back from the brink*. Ben Caldwell Labs.

Lee, N. (2019). Why celebrity, award-winning chefs are usually white men. *The Conversation*. Retrieved from https://theconversation.com/why-celebrity-award-winning-chefs-are-usually-white-men-106709

Mathieu, F., Hubble, M. A., & Miller, S. D. (2015). Burnout reconsidered: What supershrinks can teach us. *Psychotherapy Networker*. Retrieved from www.psychotherapynetworker.org/magazine/article/36/burnout-reconsidered

McKergow, M., & Pugliese, P. (Eds.) (2019). *The host leadership field book: Building engagement for performance and results*. Solution Books.

Miller, S. D., Hubble, M. A., & Chow, D. (2020). *Better results: Using deliberate practice to improve therapeutic effectiveness*. American Psychological Association.

Natynczuk, S. (2016). *Perceptions of professionalism in adventure therapy: Working towards a competency framework* [Masters Dissertation]. University of Worcester.

Natynczuk, S. (2019). Host leadership in outdoor, bush, wilderness and adventure therapy. In M. McKergow and P. Pugliese (Eds.), *The host leadership field book: Building engagement for performance and results* (pp. 42–52). Solution Books.

Natynczuk, S. (2020). Adventure therapy deconstructed: A journey towards professional practice and the good enough practitioner. *Erlebnistherapie, 2*, 10–14.

Richards, K., Hardie, A., & Anderson, N. (2020). *Outdoor mental health interventions and outdoor therapy: A statement of good practice.* Institute for Outdoor Learning. Retrieved from www.outdoor-learning.org/Good-Practice/Good-Practice/Outdoor-Mental-Health

Schwenk, E., & Natynczuk, S. (2015). Supervision and adventure therapy: Fighting burnout and providing emotional first aid for practitioners. In C. L. Norton, C. Carpenter, & A. Pryor (Eds.), *Adventure therapy around the globe: International perspectives and diverse approaches* (pp. 608–630). Common Ground.

Swindoll, S. (2000). *Day by day with Charles Swindoll.* Nelson.

9

Implementing Feedback-Informed Treatment Outdoors

"Extraordinary claims require extraordinary evidence."

Carl Sagan (1979, p. 62)

How do we know we are doing our best for our clients? We ask. Now, we know that many practitioners argue they are able to know which clients are engaged, who are at risk of dropping out of our services, or getting measurably worse, which we refer to as deterioration, but this is often guesswork. We have scholarly evidence to support this shortcoming among practitioners, no matter their level of qualification or years of experience (Chow et al., 2015), and we too are not immune. What we need is a systematic, empirically supported method for evaluating clients' experience of care. In the wise words of Carl Sagan (1979) presented above, we need to build evidence to support any claims of our own effectiveness. Though many methods for monitoring your clients' experiences exist, the simplicity of feedback-informed treatment (FIT) made this a chapter we had to include.

FIT involves the use of simple to use, reliable measures. The traditional, office-based psychotherapist will use the outcome rating scale (ORS) at the start of their session and the session rating scale (SRS) at the end. The ratings are plotted on a graph (see Appendix N) and the practitioner and client discuss any concerns to the therapeutic alliance or lack of progress.

There is nothing new about FIT. Dr. Scott D. Miller and his team at the International Center for Clinical Excellence focused on FIT since the 1990s, and this work stands on the shoulders of those before them (Miller et al., 2003, 2015, 2016). Dobud (2017) adapted Miller's work for use in expedition settings. I (Stephan) must admit feeling anxious the first time I used a post-session questionnaire overtly asking a client to rate my work. It became routine. I sometimes suspect the answers are not as honest as I would like, though I can always ask about that too. Whatever the client writes or scores

DOI: 10.4324/9781003217558-12

on their feedback form generates more co-reflection on the quality of the work and, essentially, whether they are getting what they want. It is a fair assumption that someone has turned up to therapy because they want something better.

We stated emphatically throughout this book that outdoor therapies work and work well. Despite limitations to the robustness of our evidence base, outcomes are on par to other empirically supported therapies, such as cognitive-behavioral therapy (Stigsdotter et al., 2018). However, taking adventure therapy specifically, we agree with Australian psychologists Daniel Bowen and James Neill (2013) that less than 1% of these programs undergo any formal evaluation. Additionally, when we ask outdoor therapy practitioners for the percentage of clients who have experienced clinically significant benefit, or what percent disengage from the service prematurely, or do not return after one session, we get one of two classic responses.

First, people look at us sideways. Imagine a rock climber who wants to improve their abilities without knowing how well they climb specific grades. Or a trail runner unaware of their average time for covering a certain distance. The research tells us that until practitioners know how effective they *personally* are, *not* how effective their organizations or models are, their effectiveness on average is unlikely to improve over the course of their career (Miller et al., 2020). In order to improve, practitioners must establish a baseline and know how effective they are at what they do.

And the second response we have witnessed: "The only clients who disengage are [INSERT DIAGNOSIS] ones." As we have covered, using our theories of pathology to rationalize why a person does not want to engage with us is a choice practitioners make with almost no evidence to support it.

Garcia and Weisz (2002) found most young people and their parents decide to drop out of therapy services not because of how sick they are. More often, issues in the relationship or practical barriers such as the distance required for traveling or cost of the services are the cause for concern. They discussed practitioners not listening or the receptionist shrugging off their concerns. It is these issues that often lead to ruptures in that ever important therapeutic relationship. All our education or qualifications do not really mean anything to our co-adventurers until they feel we are the right *fit*, no pun intended.

We are aware this may not be the most tantalizing of topics. Psychometrics, outcome measures, program evaluations, and outcoming monitoring are not too seductive. However, most practitioners we talk with agree that, yes, client feedback is important, but most do not engage in the practice routinely and systematically, thus building zero client-specified evidence on the efficacy of their work.

During an outdoor therapy organization's board meeting, we stressed the importance of outcome monitoring. Another researcher shared her experience of using the measures we describe below. Cursing their psychometric properties, usefulness, and their available evidence, she described the experience of interviewing past therapy clients who admitted to lying on the measures to get the therapist off their back. It is possible clients may complete the measures dishonestly. In fact, 93% of people admit lying to their therapist on at least one occasion (Shaffer, 2019). The issue with lying on a measure is not the piece of paper's dysfunction. It points to an issue in the relationship. The client is lying to *you*, not the measure. The measures we administer are not bulletproof or magic. They do not increase your effectiveness or the experiences of your co-adventurers alone. They require artful skill in administration and processing, like all things in therapy. We hope practitioners integrate feedback measures into their work to build their own evidence base and ensure the best for their co-adventurers.

With this chapter, we introduce FIT and describe its importance for therapy outdoors, being a seamless model to blend with solution-focused practices. We provide implications and ideas for monitoring client outcomes in outdoor settings, in various contexts, and finish with a discussion about how agencies can implement FIT, and develop plans for improving practitioner outcomes.

Getting FIT

Developed by researchers, clinicians, and practitioners from the International Center for Clinical Excellence, FIT is defined as a:

> pantheoretical approach for evaluating and improving the quality and effectiveness of behavioral health services. It involves routinely and formally soliciting feedback from consumers regarding the therapeutic alliance and outcome of care and using the resulting information to inform and tailor service delivery.
>
> (Bertolino et al., 2012, p. 2)

Being a *pantheoretical approach*, FIT can be implemented, and has been successfully so, in indoor and outdoor contexts, with solution-focused, trauma-informed, or psychodynamic models, in residential, outpatient, and school settings, as well as emergency rooms around the world. FIT is not just for certain practitioners. Worldwide, we have noticed more funding bodies and third party payers privilege organizations delivering such a service. SAMHSA's (2021) National Registry of Evidence-based Programs and Practices designated FIT an empirically supported treatment, due to multiple randomized clinical trials and the impact this simple, effective method has for improving psychotherapy outcomes.

Adopting this pantheoretical approach to monitoring outcomes and the client's perception of the therapeutic alliance is also important because it mitigates the impact of our respective biases. Clients typically do not arrive solution-focused, trauma-informed, or even in preference for an outdoor therapy experience. They sit across from us because of some distress in their lives, or the pressure of others has led them to external help.

I (Will) have worked with adolescents in Australia, the United States, Canada, and Norway in outdoor therapy settings. More commonly than not, these young people were not too interested in meeting at all. My role early on was to build rapport, focus on connection before correction (Selekman & Beyebach, 2014), make sure the young person felt safe, and to see what meaning they were constructing from our adventures together. If they told me something was not working, or acted out in resistance to my approach, it was *my* responsibility to change my course of action.

When working for other organizations, one issue arose when attempting to use client feedback to tailor our services. When we become feedback informed, we have to consider how seriously we are going to take the feedback we receive. When running an expedition with a group of young Indigenous women from Anangu Pitjantjatjara Yankunytjatjara (APY) Lands of remote northern South Australia, I was given feedback that the young people would have preferred a longer expedition than seven days because of the language barrier and the time it took to get accustomed to a different outdoor setting. I brought the feedback to my supervisors and program directors who turned it down. "We have always done the one week. We are not prepared to do differently."

The back half of their response was untrue. Our services were government funded, the logistics of our adventures were mostly organized by volunteers, and while we were only with our expedition groups for one week, us guides and staff remained on the property for additional days. Funding was not an issue. The lack of a feedback-informed, client-directed approach led to a decision being made that missed an opportunity to engage this young group further.

The bonus of feedback is this: if client feedback is taken seriously, and we take that feedback directly to supervisors and program directors, we get innovative. No expedition ever looks the same. With more voices, opportunities are endless. This involves, however, taking time to critically reflect on our values – and the values of those with the most at stake, the co-adventurers.

What We Value? Or What They Value?

We talk with outdoor therapy practitioners regularly about how to evaluate their services and what measures are the best to use from taking therapy to nature. For example, there is value in Russell and Gillis' (2017) Adventure Therapy Experience Scale, a measure examining the specific factors relating to adventure therapy practice, such as group adventure or time in nature. Russell et al. (2017) used the measure alongside the Outcome Questionnaire (OQ-45.2), a widely utilized outcome measure (Lambert et al., 2004), on a wilderness therapy program in Canada. While the OQ-45.2 can be utilized for your FIT practice, the instrument has 45 questions and can quickly lead to "survey fatigue" if implemented weekly as instructed. That said, Russell et al.'s (2017) initial study found that in the weeks where clients felt their adventure experience was more helpful, and when they were more mindful of their treatment aims in relation to the adventure experience, they noticed improvements to their clinical outcome. Time in nature, as a factor for predicting outcome, did not correlate with improved benefit from the adventure experience. Once again, the specific ingredients of the therapy, including being in nature, were not correlated with the success of treatment.

This is not to say the outdoor setting never contributes to outcomes, but we have to reconsider how therapy services work in relation to the setting. Remember, people typically disengage from therapy if it is 1) not working, or 2) ruptures in the therapeutic alliance exist. Said in relation to the Adventure Therapy Experience Scale, when clients felt the services they received were not only helpful, but aligned with their purpose of the therapy, the clients reported improvements in their psycho-social functioning.

So, while we are aligned to solution-focused practice in the outdoors, others may take a more ecopsychological approach, as Delaney (2020) described. We know that the specifics of our treatment, such as whether we are indoors or out, are unlikely to lead to improved outcomes (Dobud & Harper, 2018). The reason for adopting a pantheoretical approach like FIT into the outdoor therapy practice is to ensure co-adventurers are experiencing the benefit they deserve, instead of focusing on the specifics of outdoor therapy.

This is not to discredit the work of Keith Russell and Lee Gillis, as Keith's decision to use the OQ Measures in wilderness therapy, and Lee's contin-ued efforts to improve our evidence base are extraordinary. With the Ad-venture Therapy Experience Scale, these two have continued their journey with curiosity as to how this stuff works. We build on their work to ask how practitioners can know *if* it is working, not *how*. From here, we are going to examine the measures used in FIT practice and some of the strategies for adopting this work outdoors.

FIT Measures

The two widely utilized, reliable, and valid FIT measures are the Outcome Rating Scale (ORS; Miller et al., 2003) and the Session Rating Scale (SRS; Duncan et al., 2003). Both are available for practitioners to download for free in over 20 different languages, with child, young child, and group ver-sions also available. The two measures, available in the field manual, are ultra-brief, taking a client less than one minute to complete. Before going into the logistics of implementing these measures outdoors, we should look at how these measures have been utilized in traditional psychotherapy practice.

The ORS is an outcome measure of general wellbeing, which correlates well to the much longer OQ measures and others (Miller et al., 2003). The ORS is completed by the client at the start of *every therapy session*. If this is not your first session, ask the client to reflect over the previous week, or since their last session, and place a mark along each of the four 10cm lines, "each representing a different area of functioning (i.e., individual, interpersonal, social, and overall well-being" (Prescott, 2017, p. 46). As facilitator of the administration of the ORS, you can then discuss with your client what they hoped to convey with how they completed the measure. Using a ruler, mea-sure where the client checked along the lines. If they check halfway, that will be 5 points out of a possible 10.

At the tail end of your session, maybe with five minutes remaining, admin-ister the SRS, which is structured similarly to the ORS, with four 10cm lines, but measures the client's perception of the therapeutic alliance (i.e., relationality; aims and tasks; approach and method; and overall), as con-ceptualized by Bordin (1979). Upon completing this measure, invite your client to tell you about what worked, or what seemed off during the session. Remember, negative or constructive feedback helps us tailor the service. We are not interested in perfect scores, just in getting better at what we do for co-adventurers.

You can plot the scores on a graph, available when you download the measures, to track client progress. There are some important numbers to consider when interpreting the scores you receive. The ORS has a *clinical cutoff*, a boundary used to differentiate between clinical and normal ranges of distress. Based on the perfect score of 40, the clinical cutoff for adults is 25, for adolescents aged 13–18, the cutoff is 28, and for children under 13 years old, the cutoff is 32 (Miller et al., 2016). The reason for these differences is that the younger the client, the higher they tend to rate themselves.

If your client reports a score above the clinical cutoff, you should inquire about this. Maybe they were pressured to attend therapy involuntarily. In this case, it is not them with the problem, maybe it is their family members, a judge, or school counselor. We ask how the scores would change if the client completed the ORS again as if they were that person concerned with their behavior or wellbeing. We tend to see this new score, referred to as a collateral measure, drop below the cutoff. It may also be appropriate with mandated clients to use an ORS rating from the referrer. Practitioners are encouraged to use that score because you are working directly with the outcome as it relates to the original purpose of your work together. Scores above or even very close to the cutoff tend to lead to less change over time.

For example, at True North Expeditions, Inc., I (Will) have a fluctuating average intake score of 19–21, which correlates well to international averages of 19.1–19.6 for ORS intake scores (Sparks et al., 2006). Of course, some young people will arrive with scores at a 10 or lower, referred to as a statement score. They are trying to tell you something. It is important in these instances to assess the person's level of safety. You can anticipate this score will climb in subsequent sessions, but make sure to touch base with your client following the session to check in. If it stalls or deteriorates, something is wrong.

The SRS has a clinical cutoff of 36 out of 40. This means the boundary between normal ratings of the therapeutic alliance and scores to grow worried about is 36. For each factor of the SRS, you should inquire about any score below a 9 out of 10. For example, if after a rock climbing session, you receive a score of 8.5 out of 10 about the factor asking how the client rated the best hopes, aims, or topics for the session, we should check in to see what was missing. If the session did not feel as though it was aligned to that specific person's preferred future, they become less and less likely to experience that outcome.

It is helpful to practice how you will introduce the measures to your service users. If you do not take them seriously, or treat them like an administrative task, they will follow suit. If a client provides a poor SRS rating and we become defensive, we are modeling that we do not really care for their feedback. Below, we have provided a script that we have used in an expedition setting. On day one of the program, we might take a client aside and introduce the measure. This is also the perfect time to ask about their best hopes and preferred future.

> "I work a bit differently than other therapy folks. Though I know some background knowledge about what got you here, I am much more focused on making sure that you find our work together useful. I'm not the best at guessing so I hope I can create a relationship where you feel comfortable letting me know if something is off track, or if I am doing something that does not seem useful.
> "I use these two really simple pieces of paper during our work together. We will start with this one at the beginning of our trip, and then use the second after our first week together. The first one tells me how you are doing and whether or not our work is headed in the right direction. The second one looks at how you are experiencing the program, such as giving you the chance to grade our relationship, your relationship with others in the group, and if we are, in fact, working on the right stuff. Definitely not interested in wasting your time!
> "This first one, the Outcome Rating Scale, asks how you are feeling individually, interpersonally, or in your relationship with family, socially, such as how things are with school or friends, and finally an overall rating of what has been going on. All you have to do is place a tick or a check or anything along each of these four lines. The closer to the left, the lower the rating. The closer to the right, the higher. Does this make sense? Or am I rambling again?"

Put your own twist on this. Consider how you can tailor this description to the specific context of your outdoor therapy work. In Table 9.1, we outline how we have organized the administration of the ORS and SRS in various contexts.

Seeking Feedback

When it comes to seeking someone's feedback about how they perceive the quality of the therapeutic alliance, we should be mindful about how we ask these questions. Consider when you go to a restaurant and your server asks how the meal was. While you thought your salad was terrible, we often do not say so right away. Add onto this the inherent power differential between practitioner and client, it takes special consideration to establish a relationship where a client trusts you really do want to give specific, constructive

Table 9.1 Planning for FIT Implementation in Various Outdoor Therapy Settings

Specific Setting	Outcome Rating Scale	Session Rating Scale
60-minute indoor therapy session	Start of each session	End of each session
60-minute walk and talk therapy session	Start of each session	End of each session
Half or full day outdoor therapy session	Start of each session	End of each session
Overnight outdoor therapy session	Each morning	Each evening
Seven-day outdoor therapy program	Day 1, Day 3, Day 7	Day 3, Day 7
14-day outdoor therapy program	Day 1, Day 5, Day 10, Day 14	Day 5, Day 10, Day 14
Residential or longer expedition outdoor therapy program	Start of each week	End of each week

feedback. "How was everything today?" typically does not elicit anything useful. Instead, the questions we ask should be *specific* instead of general, *descriptive* not evaluative, focused on *quantities* rather than qualities, and *task-focused*, not person-oriented (Miller, 2016). Remember these questions are about our performance in our work. The server at the restaurant could ask, "Was everything the right temperature today?" At one restaurant we were thrilled to be asked, "Is there anything we could have done differently to improve your experience?" The restaurant had double booked our table and we had to wait an additional 30 minutes prior to being seated. They provided a few entrées on the house and still inquired about the experience.

How you introduce the measures and your openness to receive what could possibly be negative feedback is critical. Below, we have provided a script for introducing the SRS with a client. This example comes from an initial individual therapy session in which a young woman participated in a walk through a local park.

"Before we wrap up today, I'd like to ask if you could fill out the second form I talked about at the start of our time together today. This is called the Session Rating Scale, and basically, I use it so I can adapt and improve our work together. There is a ton of research that shows if you are enjoying our work together and feeling as though our work is focused on what matters to you that we are more likely to be successful.

"Now, remember. I am not interested in perfect scores. That means I cannot get better! [Laughter]. I am interested in your thoughts on even the smallest things that I can address – no matter how small. I promise I will not take it personally, and those fancy papers you noticed on my office wall do not mean I cannot get better. Does that make sense?"

Again, the more we stress the importance of these measures, the more those around us will as well. Beyond the measures, the real magic of FIT is what we do with the information we receive. This means we must have our eye on the big picture research about what certain scores or trends mean, and also spend time focusing on how we respond to the scores and feedback we receive.

Building the Culture of Feedback

Billy was on a 14-day expedition in the Australian bush when, on day 5, his trip leader, a social worker who was being observed by a social work student on field placement, took Billy away from the group of ten other young adult participants to administer the ORS and the Group Session Rating Scale. Billy's ORS rating improved by 5 points, but the group session rating was below the clinical cutoff at a 33. When asked about this, Billy said he was in the wrong group. He did not get along with the other participants, yet really engaged with the staff, especially the social work student. The three talked about this and organized time each day when Billy could have time away from the group, doing something fun with the social work student. Billy said, "That will be awesome!" Not only did the alliance rating improve, so did Billy's outcome. After completing her master's in social work, the newly graduated social worker continued working with Billy and his reported well-being climbed. He felt he was in the right place.

I (Will) was the social worker sitting next to that social work student. I could have received Billy's feedback defensively. I could have been a gatekeeper to the student I supervised and said she was not ready to work individually with a client such as Billy. Maybe I should have thought about the group; Billy volunteered to attend a group expedition but did not like the other participants. Should he just "get over it?" I chose to instead privilege Billy's feedback, knowing by not doing so I could very well be gatekeeping Billy from the experience he deserved. It was not about me; it was about Billy's experience and privileging it.

Many agencies worldwide engage in FIT. Many practitioners have an enthusiastic colleague or boss who tells them to get engaged with the measures, and they may reluctantly start doing it. Then, practitioners may not see the benefit and stop. The issue is here, and what makes implementation challenging, is that we need to go beyond the measures (Miller et al., 2015). What we do with the data and the feedback we receive is most important.

Below, we have provided a few key points and a case vignette to describe what we can do with specific feedback we receive. We have found what clients describe are often smaller rather than larger issues. The little things, like what time of day we meet, or how far we hike, can be more difficult to change when accommodating large groups or organizational restraints because of complexities around group dynamics or scheduling with others outside the expedition, such as people providing transport or expecting us to turn up at a specific time and place.

We acknowledge there is too much information for us to present in this one chapter, so we created a table for use while working outdoors (see Appendix O). Still, we recommend looking at the FIT literature presented throughout and included in the reference list. Before concluding this chapter, we provide some strategies for using the FIT measures in natural environments.

Interpreting Intake Scores

What is most important is that we obtain an accurate reading of a person's reported wellbeing before beginning our adventure. The initial ORS score is the reference point we use for interpreting all subsequent ORS administrations. When we receive an initial ORS score well below the clinical cutoff, we can expect the client to report change earlier rather than later. Someone reporting a higher level of distress is more likely to experience greater amounts of change on the ORS. If their score is closer to the clinical cutoff, or above, the amount and speed at which changes occur is less than those with lower scores. In both cases, we need to discuss how our client constructs meaning around their ORS scores. If their score is close to the cutoff, but they are seeking our help for a specific reason, such as a phobia, we should focus solely on their preference for seeking our services. If we focus on areas of their life outside of their best hopes for our work together, they risk deterioration.

ORS Scores above the Clinical Cutoff

Intake scores falling above the clinical cutoff are a warning sign for practitioners. People with very high intake scores tend to drop. Scores above the cutoff can be common for mandated clients or those young in age. In this case, we need to inquire about an outcome rating in relation to why they are there or ask a client's caregiver to complete an outcome rating as well for a collateral score. This is not to discount the client's perception of their wellbeing, but to obtain an appropriate measure relating to what brings them to therapy.

Riley was referred for outdoor therapy after numerous therapy experiences did not elicit his parents' preferred outcome of reducing his substance use and improving school attendance. When Riley completed his initial outcome rating, he scored a 36 of a possible 40, well above the cutoff of 28 for a teenager like himself. Upon asking about what brought him to the session, he talked about recent fights with his mother, who believed he had a drug problem. The practitioner asked Riley how his mother would complete the measure if she were present. The score was now a 19. The practitioner asked about the discrepancy in scores saying, "I wonder if these scores were closer together if there would be fewer arguments at home." The two agreed to use both Riley's individual ORS rating and the collateral measure, which was closely linked to why Riley was engaged in the service, and worked together to improve the family conflict in Riley's life, which subsequently led to reductions in substance use.

Alliance Scores below the Clinical Cutoff

A low alliance score is a gift. Seriously! Research actually indicates that alliance scores that go from bad (<36) to good (39–40) are amazing predictors of effective therapy (Owen et al., 2016). While 75% of clients will typically score above the clinical cutoff of 36 for SRS, initial scores coming in below 36 are hopeful indicators. First, it lets you know that your client felt safe enough to tell you something was missing or off track. Second, it provides you the opportunity to use the person's negative feedback to tailor the service. What you do with the feedback is most important.

We must inquire as to what was missing during the session or the period of time in residential or expedition programming. Again, it is good to avoid "why questions" here. Seeking negative feedback is hard. Consider the previous example of the unsatisfying salad; most of us are uncomfortable giving our honest opinion and instead leave the restaurant only to go home and post it online anonymously. Further, most are not very good at asking for this feedback. The server typically asks, "How was everything?" while your mouth is full of our last bite of beef wellington. You say, "Everything is fine," and when the server walks away roll your eyes at your friends while venting on your drive home how slow the drinks service was and the temperature of your entrées. We must ask questions specific to our performance, in relation to SRS scores.

Imagine after four days on expedition, a co-adventurer scores a 9 or above in the areas of your relational bond and liking your outdoor approach, but a 6 out of 10 in the domain of goals and topics. This could indicate that despite having a good time on the program, we might not be working with their best hopes or addressing the context of what brought them to the program in the first place. You might say, "So it seems like something was missing in relation to the purpose of our work together. If I could lead those four days over again, what could I have done to make this more tailored to your best hopes for being here?" It is important not to ask too many questions, as we do not want people to feel interrogated. More important are specific questions:

- What can you do more or less of?
- Are there certain people the client could benefit from having more time with?
- What activities have worked, and which did not? Which could we have more of?
- Thank them for any information you give and remind them that you are always aiming to get better at your work. Life is not perfect, and neither are you.

During our consultation work with various agencies, we are often asked how practitioners can navigate the negative feedback they receive. Some feel anxious or worried that negative feedback is indicative of their overall effectiveness. Be reminded that the most effective practitioners are *better* at eliciting negative feedback early on in care (Owen et al., 2016). Second, if you did not obtain the feedback, the opportunity to reassess your game plan and tailor your service becomes harder. Finally, we hear apprehension about using the measures to assess people's experiences as practitioners believe they are equipped to assess the client progress and alliance ratings without the use of measures. Unfortunately, the data indicate otherwise (Hannan et al., 2005).

We do not prefer the use of numbers as some reductionistic philosophical stance. Instead, they remind us of a series of patterns and algorithms to help us to check our biases and remain focused on clients' best hopes and their experience in our care. For example, after obtaining the initial alliance rating, any drop in alliance score, even by one point, is a warning sign for future dropout (Miller et al., 2016). These small changes are harder to catch without the numbers to help. Aligned with our philosophical underpinnings of social construction, described in Chapter 3, we view the numbers similarly to Tilsen and McNamee (2015) who argue FIT is the very place evidence-based practice meets social construction.

A Lack of Early Change

Despite arguments about brief versus long-term therapy, successful experiences in therapy are typically privy to early change. Howard et al. (1993, 1996) argued that early change makes sense as this will improve a therapy recipient's hope that this course of treatment will work. This, in turn, reduces the likelihood the client disengages from the service. Remember, co-adventurers can still drop out in residential or expedition settings where they cannot physically leave the program. They drop out emotionally and are simply along for the ride. Below, we have outlined some considerations for practitioners experiencing a lack of early change in their service.

Informed by psychotherapy dose effect data, Bertolino et al. (2012) advised FIT adopters that 30% of clients demonstrate measurable improvement by the second session, 60–65% by the seventh session, and 70–75% after six months. After one year, 85% of clients improve. While every individual's therapy experience is different, the early reporting of benefit is a strong indicator for the overall outcome. Thus, we must be mindful of examining the client's experience of outcome from session one, no matter the type of therapy we deliver.

During my (Will) doctoral research, I interviewed a young woman who was securely transported involuntarily to a wilderness therapy program in the United States. After months in the program, her therapist left and she was assigned a new practitioner. The new therapist validated how difficult her experience had been thus far and communicated empathy surrounding the transport experience and her traumatic family dynamics. This changed her experience. She engaged with the new therapist, though did not have as much time with him as she preferred. Had this program monitored her outcome and alliance ratings, change could have occurred sooner rather than later. This would have been an evidence-based decision. Instead, she left demoralized and upset about her more than 90-day experience in the woods (Dobud, 2020).

Conclusion: Failing Successfully

When we have a client's outcome and alliance data available, the evidence is used to inform our decision making, hence being *evidence-informed*. This data includes what we know about therapy outcome research, client feedback, and the numbers associated with their outcome. If having frank conversations with a co-adventurer about the lack of progress or deteriorating alliance ratings, supervision, and attempts to adjust the course of our work do not lead to progress, it is time to consider *failing successfully* (Valla & Prescott, 2019). This we owe to those whom we serve.

Our work will not be effective for everyone. We use FIT to know who is falling through the cracks so we can adjust our services to best meet their needs. If we have worked with someone for more than eight sessions, or a few weeks of residential care, and the numbers are telling us we are not improving, we consider a referral to another practitioner. We avoid blaming the client, instead describing that there are times when two people are not the best fit. We explain they should experience benefits early on to calm the nerves that they must start the process all over again. In one scenario, I (Will) referred a client to a colleague of mine at a local mental health clinic. I had seen the young adult for nearly six months and despite early change, his outcome rating was slowly dropping. We met with his mother on two occasions, and we made the decision to try help elsewhere. To be frank, I told them that I did not want to waste their time. He saw the colleague for four sessions, over the course of three weeks, and re-enrolled in trade school and completed a plumbing qualification.

What made my failure "successful" is in how I initiated our relationship and also how I ended it. From the beginning, I let the client and mother know that I will be monitoring outcome and alliance throughout the course of care. If there is something that seems off, I would let them know. It did not come as a shock when we sat down to look at the charts. He liked our hikes and fishing trips but did not feel any more motivation to get out of bed each day. Despite attempts to change the dose or focus of our sessions, nothing budged. The client did seem disappointed, and I asked him to call me and let me know how he felt with the new therapist. He enjoyed the first session.

It can be intimidating to refer our stuck cases to our friends and colleagues. We recommend building a network of likeminded practitioners in your area; people you feel comfortable asking for advice and discussing the areas in your practice requiring some attention. We all have them. This makes failing a bit less scary.

A few months passed and I received a bouquet of native Australian flowers at my front gate. I am not used to thank you gifts at our practice. I was caught off guard. It was from the client's mother. The note inside read: "Thank you for saving our son." I called her and we laughed on the phone. I actually failed! She told me she had such little hope that the mental health system could actually help, as nothing had worked before. She shared that she has a refreshing view of the "good people out there doing good and honest work." I thanked her for the kind words, and we have not spoken since. That said, a few times each year a mother calls me and says, "I have heard you can help my child. Donna told me you do amazing work." This has continued since 2013.

Failing successfully is not an abstract colloquialism. It is an expression of honesty, transparency, humility, and how we act in the best interest of our co-adventurers. Consider your game plan for failing successfully. Just like our evacuation plan when handling an injury outdoors, what will you do when the numbers are not falling in your favor? Failing successfully kept our practices open and thriving. There is no "bad outcome" when we help those we work with get to a more appropriately tailored service. That said, there are things we can do along the way to critically reflect on the work we are doing. This involves the reigniting of supervision, which we discuss in the following chapter.

References

Bertolino, B., Bargmann, S., & Miller, S. D. (2012). *Manual 1: What works in therapy: A primer*. International Center for Clinical Excellence.

Bordin, E. S. (1979). The generalizability of the psychoanalytic concept of the working alliance. *Psychotherapy: Theory, Research & Practice, 16*(3), 1–9.

Bowen, D. J., & Neill, J. T. (2013). A meta-analysis of adventure therapy outcomes and moderators. *The Open Psychology Journal, 6*, Article 28-53. https://doi.org/10.2174/1874350120130802001

Chow, D. L., Miller, S. D., Seidel, J. A., Kane, R. T., Thornton, J. A., & Andrews, W. P. (2015). The role of deliberate practice in the development of highly effective psychotherapists. *Psychotherapy, 52*(3), 337–345. https://doi.org/10.1037/pst0000015

Delaney, M. E. (2020). Ecopsychological approaches to therapy. In N. J. Harper & W. W. Dobud (Eds.), *Outdoor Therapies* (pp. 30–41). Routledge.

Dobud, W. W. (2017). Towards an evidence-informed adventure therapy: Implementing feedback-informed treatment in the field. *Journal of Evidence-Informed Social Work*, 14(3), 172–182. https://doi.org/10.1080/23761407.2017.1304310

Dobud, W. W. (2020). *Experiences of adventure therapy: A narrative inquiry* [Doctoral Dissertation]. Charles Sturt University.

Dobud, W. W., & Harper, N. J. (2018). Of dodo birds and common factors: A scoping review of direct comparison trials in adventure therapy. *Complementary Therapies in Clinical Practice*, 31, 16–24. https://doi.org/10.1016/j.ctcp.2018.01.005

Duncan, B. L., Miller, S. D., Sparks, J. A., Claud, D. A., Reynolds, L. R., Brown, J., & Johnson, L. D. (2003). The Session Rating Scale: Preliminary psychometric properties of a "working" alliance measure. *Journal of Brief Therapy*, 3(1), 3–12.

Garcia, J. A., & Weisz, J. R. (2002). When youth mental health care stops: Therapeutic relationship problems and other reasons for ending youth outpatient treatment. *Journal of Consulting and Clinical Psychology*, 70(2), 439–443. https://doi.org/10.1037/0022-006X.70.2.439

Hannan, C., Lambert, M. J., Harmon, C., Nielsen, S. L., Smart, D. W., Shimokawa, K., et al. (2005). A lab test and algorithms for identifying clients at risk for treatment failure. *Journal of Clinical Psychology: In Session*, 61, 155–163. https://doi.org/10.1002/jclp.20108

Howard, K. I., Lueger, R. J., Maling, M. S., & Martinovich, Z. (1993). A phase model of psychotherapy outcome: Causal mediation of change. *Journal of Consulting and Clinical Psychology*, 61(4), 678–685. https://doi.org/10.1037/0022-006X.61.4.678

Howard, K. I., Moras, K., Brill, P. L., Martinovich, Z., & Lutz, W. (1996). Evaluation of psychotherapy: Efficacy, effectiveness, and patient progress. *American Psychologist*, 51(10), 1059–1064. https://doi.org/10.1037/0003-066X.51.10.1059

Lambert, M. J., Gregersen, A. T., & Burlingame, G. M. (2004). The Outcome Questionnaire-45. In M. E. Maruish (Ed.), *The use of psychological testing for treatment planning and outcomes assessment: Instruments for adults* (pp. 191–234). Lawrence Erlbaum Associates Publishers.

Miller, S. D. (2016). *What is the essential quality of effective feedback? New research points the way*. Retrieved from scottdmiller.com/essential-quality-of-effective-feedback/

Miller, S. D., Bargmann, S., Chow, D., Seidel, J., & Maeschalck, C. (2016). Feedback-informed treatment (FIT): Improving the outcome of psychotherapy one person at a time. In W. O'Donohue & A. Maragakis (Eds.), *Quality improvement in behavioral health* (pp. 247–262). Springer International Publishing. https://doi.org/10.1007/978-3-319-26209-3_16

Miller, S. D., Duncan, B. L., Brown, J., Sparks, J. A., & Claud, D. A. (2003). The outcome rating scale: A preliminary study of the reliability, validity, and feasibility of a brief visual analog measure. *Journal of Brief Therapy, 2*(2), 91–100.

Miller, S. D., Hubble, M. A., & Chow, D. (2020). *Better results: Using deliberate practice to improve therapeutic effectiveness.* American Psychological Association.

Miller, S. D., Hubble, M. A., Chow, D., & Seidel, J. (2015). Beyond measures and monitoring: Realizing the potential of feedback-informed treatment. *Psychotherapy, 52*(4), 449–457. https://doi.org/10.1037/pst0000031

Owen, J., Miller, S. D., Seidel, J., & Chow, D. (2016). The working alliance in treatment of military adolescents. *Journal of Consulting and Clinical Psychology, 84*(3), 200–210. https://doi.org/10.1037/ccp0000035

Prescott, D. S. (2017). Feedback-informed treatment: An overview of the basics and core competencies. In D. S. Prescott, C. L. Maeschalck, & S. D. Miller (Eds.), *Feedback-informed treatment in clinical practice: Reaching for excellence* (pp. 37–52). American Psychological Association. https://doi.org/10.1037/0000039-003

Russell, K. C., & Gillis, H. L. (2017). The adventure therapy experience scale: The psychometric properties of a scale to measure the unique factors moderating an adventure therapy experience. *Journal of Experiential Education, 40*(2), 135–152. https://doi.org/10.1177%2F1053825917690541

Russell, K. C., Gillis, H. L., & Kivlighan, D. M., Jr. (2017). Process factors explaining psycho-social outcomes in adventure therapy. *Psychotherapy, 54*(3), 273–280. https://doi.org/10.1037/pst0000131

Sagan, C. (1979). *Broca's brain: Reflections on the romance of science.* Random House Digital, Inc.

Selekman, M. D., & Beyebach, M. (2014). *Changing self-destructive habits: Pathways to solutions with couples and families.* Routledge.

Shaffer, A. (2019). The truth about lies: Almost all patients tell some lies while in therapy: But what patients keep hidden might reveal more than therapists think. *Monitor on Psychology, 50*(5), 38. Retrieved from: www.apa.org/monitor/2019/05/truth-lies

Sparks, J. A., Miller, S. D., Bohanske, R. T., & Claud, D. A. (2006). Giving youth a voice: A preliminary study of the reliability and validity of a brief outcome measure for children, adolescents, and caretakers. *Journal of Brief Therapy, 5*, 66–82.

Stigsdotter, U. K., Corazon, S. S., Sidenius, U., Nyed, P. K., Larsen, H. B., & Fjorback, L. O. (2018). Efficacy of nature-based therapy for individuals with stress-related illnesses: Randomised controlled trial. *The British Journal of Psychiatry, 213*(1), 404–411. https://doi.org/10.1192/bjp.2018.2

Substance Abuse and Mental Health Services Administration [SAMHSA]. (2021). *SAMHSA – Substance Abuse and Mental Health Services Administration*. Retrieved from www.samhsa.gov/

Tilsen, J., & McNamee, S. (2015). Feedback informed treatment: Evidence-based practice meets social construction. *Family Process, 54*(1), 124–137. https://doi. org/10.1111/famp.12111

Valla, B., & Prescott, D. S. (2019). *Beyond best practice: How mental health services can be better*. Routledge.

10
Re-Igniting Supervision in Outdoor Therapy

"Better we raise our skill than lower the climb."
Royal Robbins (1994, p. 62)

Supervision can be neglected. Requirements for the supervision of therapists and practitioners vary throughout the world, and at times, outdoor practitioners may not understand the benefits of supervision, conflating it with management, which should remain distinct from clinical or counseling supervision. One type of supervision is about your professional therapeutic work with clients, the other is about how you fit in with corporate culture and your prospects for ongoing employment. The difference is fundamental. We expand on what supervision means for us, and its importance in this chapter.

In some states, and this is across the world, supervision is only required for therapists or counselors in training. In others, ongoing supervision is a requirement of continuing professional practice. I (Stephan) have been advocating for supervision in outdoor and adventure therapy since it showed up as the "Elephant in the Room" at the 2009 International Adventure Therapy Conference (IATC), the theme of which was professional practice: "Towards a Profession," encouraging practitioners to critically evaluate their industry and its approach to, and place within, psychological therapy. Two of us seemed to notice that no-one was talking about supervision. At the time, the late and dearly missed Dr. Elspeth Schwenk was on the board of trustees for the British Association for Counselling and Psychotherapy and on her way to becoming deputy chair, a professional counselor and supervisor with a thriving private practice. Elspeth and I got together and wrote a paper on supervision, fighting burnout, and providing emotional first aid specifically for adventure therapy practitioners (Schwenk & Natynczuk, 2015), which we presented at the following IATC in the Czech Republic in 2012 and again as

DOI: 10.4324/9781003217558-13

a workshop at the IATC in 2015 in Denver. In between, we went on a little mission presenting our ideas about the usefulness of supervision at a handful of conferences and workshops.

Good supervision is essential to maintaining the wellbeing of both the practitioners and those they serve. A trained supervisor will have an eye on ethical practice and a model for the supervision they offer, and there are quite a few to choose from, though not as many as there are talking therapies. A useful model considers the web of relationships, and quality of practice and professionalism impacting on any practitioner's work. Elements of coaching and mentoring also come into supervision, though little if any counseling as that is something entirely different. Before we examine models for supervision useful for our work, we describe some of the current issues with supervising, not only therapy practice, but therapy outdoors.

If It's Broken, Fix It

Most therapy experiences occur behind closed doors. Taking this work to the outdoors means our practice undergoes even less observation. Put bluntly, it is quite possible those working with individuals outside will hardly ever have their work observed (Dobud & Cavanaugh, 2020). Not only does this mean outdoor therapy practitioners become solely responsible for maintaining their co-adventurers' physical safety, such as tying the appropriate knot at the right time, but ensuring their therapeutic work is safe and effective. Supervision for outdoor practitioners should explore the blending of active bodily engagement and talking therapy, and ensure the practice is ethical and where legislation exists, legal. That is asking a lot from a supervisor able to work effectively with an outdoor therapy practitioner.

Therapy is more art than medicine. Imagine one of us writing a song on the guitar in the key of E flat minor with an upbeat tempo in 3/4 time. Maybe you will be able to read the lyrics or see the chord progressions, but will you ever be able to interpret the song without actually hearing it? After all, and we all know this inherently, two different guitar players and vocalists are going to perform this specific song very differently. This is a metaphor for one of the major problems with clinical counseling supervision.

In the outdoors, we might be on a multi-day expedition with a group, and only a satellite phone call could connect us to a clinical supervisor. What are we able to relay to our supervisor and how might our assessment of a client's experience be interpreted by the supervisor? In a nutshell, it is no wonder that worldwide, clinical supervision contributes little to no variance in improving therapeutic outcomes (Caldwell, 2015). It is no different than trying to recall what happened on a first date, or during our first kayak journey down a class three rapid. All we have is one person's interpretation, and good supervision needs some real-time observation.

Many therapeutic practitioners will tell you supervision is essential to their professional development (Miller et al., 2020). The data indicate otherwise. Watkins Jr. (2011) used the available data to conclude that: "We do not seem any more able to say now (as opposed to 30 years ago) that psychotherapy supervision contributes to patient outcome" (p. 235). We have ideas for why this is.

In Chapter 2, we constructed an argument for basing your outdoor practice on the best available evidence to inform how to be most effective in your work, and how to get better at doing it. In Chapter 9, feedback-informed treatment was presented as a means for building your evidence, using empirically supported strategies to improve your co-adventurers' experiences. What we do with this information is important when we consider how we or others supervise outdoor therapy practices. In the following two sections, we will describe two issues: 1) the lack of client voice; and 2) the importance of bringing data to supervision.

Client Voice

When in a stuck place with a client, there are many avenues available to receive clinical support. We can book a session with our supervisor, phone a friend, or post a question on the many outdoor or adventure therapy social media pages, of course while respecting client confidentiality. All might be useful, but the inherent limitation is in how we bring our client's preferences to the supervision meeting.

We avoid gossiping, diagnosing, and over-theorizing why certain people make a lack of progress in our care, or blaming the client for their disengagement. A general rule is to spend less than three minutes, or even 90 seconds, describing what the issue is (Bargmann, 2017). The more we talk about the case, the more our assessment and bias interferes with our understanding of the client's engagement or lack of progress. After all, it might be our conceptualization getting in the way. Focus discussion with your supervisor on barriers to engagement or outcome that may be the result of the practitioner's actions.

During a recent group consultation with a trauma-informed outdoor therapy agency, one of the youth workers described an issue relating to a participant's engagement. They had gone on a few short hikes, and upon scheduling a full-day rock climbing session, the young person would not leave their bedroom. She described how the participant's early adversities and complex trauma were interfering with their engagement. Instead of focusing on the trauma, we inquired about what the client wants from their relationship. This was a hard question to answer. If we do not know, we are navigating with a compass needle not pointing north. The youth worker scheduled a phone call with the participant and sought the reasons for missing the longer days. With support from the peer supervision group, we remained open and transparent, did not communicate defensiveness, and listened for the client's preferences. He did not want to go rock climbing and felt he only had to agree to go to please the worker. She focused subsequent supervision sessions on questions she could ask her co-adventurers to obtain their best hopes for their work together.

Implementing mechanisms for gathering client voice about progress, or lack thereof, the quality of your relationship, and the importance of your work together is important. We have created a progress report, completed between the practitioner and co-adventurer collaboratively, that practitioners are encouraged to use in supervision (see Appendix P). If their alliance scores deteriorate, we ask for honest feedback so we can make necessary adjustments. If our work together continues to stall, we seek supervision and describe the issues based on what the client is telling us. We never say anything about co-adventurers we would not say to their face.

Using the progress report to gather more client voices can feel very different to participants who have experienced numerous therapy failures. Marginalized and disadvantaged populations may be wary of professionals, such as social workers or juvenile justice workers, and it can take work to communicate that you only care about making their experience meaningful and useful.

Harry, an Indigenous young person in Canada, was removed from home and placed into residential care facilities at eight years old. The workers in his life were transient and burnt out. When offered to engage in an outdoor therapy, Harry was certain this was just a punishment for his bad behavior. "They just want to control me! Typical fucking white people," he said. The worker assured him this was not the case and continued to ask for Harry's best hopes, of which he was adamant there were none. At the third session, the practitioner asked Harry to complete the progress note. Cleverly, the practitioner said, "I like to fill this out to help me get better at my job.

Though I'm experienced and have some training, I'm still learning from people I meet and would love your help by completing this progress note with me." Harry described that he liked her more than he thought he would and felt happier most of the time, though he really wanted to focus more on mastering one adventurous activity instead of doing a different one each time. The worker asked what difference it would make, and Harry described having never been skilled at anything. His feedback was taken on board and their work blossomed.

Being Driven by Data

Evidence-informed practitioners base their practice on the best available evidence around how therapy works and the evidence they build throughout their practice. As feedback-informed providers, we understand how the data we collect using the ORS and SRS can help us to tailor our work and provide clues when in stuck situations. While it is important to metaphorically bring your co-adventurers into supervision, we encourage you to use the data, the numbers, to help paint the picture of what is going on.

As social constructionists, it may sound strange that we stress using quantitative measures to assess client progress. Numbers help us to check our biases. We might think a co-adventurer's trajectory is aiming upwards, or think highly of the quality of our relationship, yet on the measure they tell us otherwise. When training practitioners on using the FIT measures, the most common apprehension is whether it will change how they want to work (the practitioner's preference), whether it measures what they think is most important (the practitioner's value), or that the practitioner might find out information they do not want to hear (again, the practitioner's issue). Bringing numbers to supervision helps ensure the client's perception of outcome and the alliance are documented.

A note on the philosophical underpinnings of FIT. Advocates for the decolonization of mental and behavioral health services and education have voiced concern that quantitative methods are the tool of the colonist. As advocates of decolonizing our work (see Natynczuk & Dobud, 2021), we acknowledge and stress the acceptance of varying worldviews. In fact, we firmly believe gathering data in relation to client voice, not simply on topics we value, such as time in nature, is essential to decenter the practitioner, thus avoiding colonizing another's experience, leaving no trace. When we have a session we find incredible, yet the client finds it meaningless, we want to know. Numbers help. Because FIT has been rolled out around the world, we have clues and hints based on the numbers to help us when things are going off the rails.

Below is a case example from an outdoor therapy expedition using the format of our progress report. The practitioner, a licensed clinical social worker named Sally, scheduled a call with us to review the progress on day 9 of their 21-day expedition. The call was held at night, away from the group while the participants were asleep. The case example is informed by the work of Bargmann (2017), and a blank version of Table 10.1 is included in the field manual for your use (see Appendix Q). We instructed Sally to adopt the following case presentation: 1) Name; 2) Age; 3) Gender identity; 4) Relationship status/family; 5) Work/education; 6) Concerns of the client/significant others; 7) Treatment start; 8) Current treatment (including medication); 9) Previous treatment; 10) Abuse; 11) Reason for seeking treatment. After the case presentation, the supervisor invites the practitioner to share the outcome data and focuses on the quality of the therapeutic alliance using the data from the SRS.

Case Example

The format of the supervision section is presented in Appendix R. After gathering the data and hearing the case presentation, we brainstormed ways the practitioner could talk with Steve about making the most of their time together, given the low rating in relation to his purpose for being on the program and lack of engagement in what they were doing together. Most important is that the practitioner leaves supervision feeling capable, confident, affirmed in their practice, and able to take a refreshed look at their work. We agreed that the group processes or scheduled "therapy time" were not working. Doing more was contraindicated. We reflected on the case presentation and outcome data, asking Sally if anything stood out. She noticed that this program could turn out like every other therapeutic intervention Steve had endured; lots of busy work and no outcome. She agreed to sit with Steve the next day, away from the group, and validate his sense of being couch surfed from therapist to therapist. She would revisit with Steve how outdoor therapy can work and explore his best hopes for the future.

While meeting away from the group, Steve spoke about his mother for the first time. Sally did not direct this interaction, but as she asked about Steve's best hopes, he opened up. He said most therapists just focus on her passing and it always felt fake because they did not really care about who he was. The effort of sitting with Steve away from the group demonstrated relational

Table 10.1 Format for Evidence-Informed Supervision Outdoors

Case Presentation	
Name: Steve	**Age:** 17
Gender identity: Male	
Relationship/family: Single, lives with single father, mother passed away due to suicide, younger brother	
Work/education: Full time high school student, works part time at a sports store	
Treatment start: 9 days ago	**Current treatment:** 21-day wilderness therapy expedition. No medication.
Previous treatment: Has seen numerous therapists. He says they just ask stupid questions and seem very "stereotypical." Only goes because his father makes him.	
Abuse: None	
Reasons for seeking treatment: His father made him go on the expedition due to issues at home. Father's concerns are related to school engagement, marijuana use, and dealing with the loss of Steve's mother.	
Outcome Data	
First ORS score: 21.5/40	**Last ORS score:** 22.3/40
Quality of the Therapeutic Alliance	
First SRS score: 32/40	**Last SRS score:** 34/40
Relational bond: Steve says he likes the people on the program. Feels like he trusts the staff and other participants. Rates this section high.	
Best hopes/purpose: Steve says he is only here to get his father off his back. Says nothing will help and just wants to move out and be independent.	
Means/methods: Steve likes camping but does not engage with journaling or group processes. Likes joking with other participants but avoids any therapeutic work.	

care for who he was, not simply trying to explore his grief and loss. Steve's outcome rating increased, and he reported hope that Sally was someone who could help. After the program, Sally reflected with us on what went well, what she could do better next time, and how she could practice her interpersonal skills in preparation for her next expedition.

Ideally, this process can take 15–20 minutes (Bargmann, 2017). We spent little time on the case presentation and dived directly into the data and client voice. Given Steve and Sally were on expedition together for 11 more days, we agreed that a follow-up call with Sally would be useful at the next opportunity. Steve's outcome rating increased before the next meeting, and his alliance rating was above the clinical cutoff. After the expedition, Sally developed a plan for further professional development in contracting with young people about the purpose of their work together.

Data and client voice inform our supervision. We also require some theoretical frameworks to inform what we talk about and why. In the section that follows, we examine some of the supervision models we have utilized and their versatility in the outdoors. Just like psychotherapy models, there are too many of them and they all tend to work the same. Unless practitioners become data-driven in their supervision framework, there is a high risk that simply adopting these models will not correlate with improved outcomes for co-adventurers.

Some Theoretical Frameworks for Supervision Models

The supervision models we have found most useful during our professional development are briefly mentioned below. Anyone seeking to know more is recommended to go to original references and read further, including the criticisms. Our purpose here is to report that theoretical frameworks exist for supervision, and any trained supervisor should know what you are talking about when you enquire as to what informs their supervision practice, referring to models they might have adopted. As you will see, there are many approaches to take on board and at least as many criticisms. We can only suggest that you take an informed choice about what adds to useful supervision for your own work. We will outline a few of our favorite models below, just to bring them to your attention and to show that supervision, like counseling, should be informed by theoretical considerations.

Supervision models are framed to help you get the most from your supervisor-practitioner relationship. For example, Inskipp and Proctor's (2001) *Functional Model* and Hawkins' and Shohet's (2009) *Seven-Eyed Model* examine what influences a practitioner's work, such as what people other than the client might want from the therapy, the interested stakeholders, and the inappropriate challenges complicating a co-adventurer's experience, such as power play in an organization. We tend to blend these two models in a person-centered approach. Other models, such as Page and Wosket's (2001) *Cyclical Model* and Carroll's (1996) *Seven Generic Tasks*, while kept in the background, also inform our practice. Many supervision models overlap or draw on each other in development. While Abiddin (2008) gave comprehensive reviews of supervision models, Davys and Beddoe (2010) found little consensus on what constitutes good supervision. This is a challenge for our field. For us in writing this chapter, this is part of the reason supervision is not always valued as a component of good practice. Our approach has been to borrow what is most helpful to the practitioner's situation, practice, strengths, outcome data, and best hopes.

The attraction of Hawkins' and Shohet's (2009) *Seven-Eyed Model* is its comprehensiveness. Not only is it applicable to counseling supervision, it applies to a range and variety of allied professions, such as coaching (Hawkins & Schwenk, 2010). Perhaps the overwhelming lesson from supervision models is the extent to which supervision belongs to a web of responsibility and accountability, a sort of counseling ecology of interdependency for all directly, and indirectly, involved in the therapeutic practice.

Hawkins and Shohet (2009) used the term *matrix* to describe the extension of the practitioner-client relationship through to the organization and processes feeding into the supervisor-practitioner-client relationship. Ethics remain at the center in all of this. A model that keeps us mindful of the web of responsibilities is relevant to outdoor therapy practice, holding the wider picture in mind. Importantly, Hawkins and Shohet (2009) draw attention to cultural neutrality and remain independent of counseling modalities, supervision styles, or developmental stages. This sounds reminiscent of aspects of host leadership. While their model presents as complex in diagrammatic form, the areas of focus are clear enough. These are briefly:

- Focus on the practitioner's clients and what and how they present
- Exploration of the strategies and interventions used by the supervised
- Exploration of the relationship between the client and the supervised
- Focus on the supervised
- Focus on the supervisory relationship
- The supervisor focusses on their own process
- Focus on the wider contexts in which the work happens.

(Hawkins & Shohet, 2009, pp. 83–84)

The main intention is to allow the supervisor to move between areas of focus and gain clarity about the strengths and weaknesses of their own style. Done well, little is avoided or missed in the process. Self-knowledge on how one influences the supervision processes maintains objectivity, honesty, integrity, fairness, and robustness (Žorga, 2007). Knowing the model also equips the practitioner with a language to appraise, negotiate, and review their supervision (Hawkins & Shohet, 2009), becoming good practice for avoiding a power play in the supervisor-practitioner relationship (Kaberry, 2000).

Hawkins and Shohet (2009) acknowledged the major criticisms of their model. Opponents find their work hierarchical, less than integrative, and somewhat inverted – the wider context should be contained within the other aspects or modes. However, the *Seven-Eyed Model* has been in use since 1985 and appears generally robust and useful across cultures, professions, and therapies despite criticism for its complexity (Aten et al., 2008).

The Inskipp and Proctor (1990) *Functional Model* drew on Egan's (2002) 3-Stage Helper Model, itself presented in an updated form. The model's emphasis on *Normative, Formative,* and *Restorative* is particularly effective for shaping the broad structure of a supervision session and addresses the *ethical practitioner,* the *competent practitioner,* and the *confident and creative practitioner,* respectively. However, O'Donovan et al. (2011) argued supervision as currently practiced is not so effective in its normative function. The restorative function in Inskipp and Proctor's model is important to the way we work, and relevant to avoiding burnout. Practitioners can benefit from a good vent of frustrations and then, in exploring their practice from a strengths-based perspective, gain a degree of restoration and affirmation for the good things they do.

Egan's (2002) work informed several models of supervision (e.g., Newnham-Kanas et al., 2010), yet has been criticized as being prescriptive, mechanical, overly masculine, and cumbersome in its use of language (Wosket, 2006). Like all theories for therapeutic change, Egan (2002) recognized his model lacked some universal appeal. In terms of its direct applicability to supervision, there were limited distinctions between counseling and supervision, which Shulman (2006) identified as modeling poor practice.

Page and Wosket's (2001) *Cyclical Model* is more complex with five stages further subdivided into five segments. The initial stages to 1) *Contract;* 2) *Focus;* 3) *Space;* 4) *Bridge;* and then 5) *Review* can work well as a general guide, though the 25 subdivisions seem to be unwieldy. This model also draws on Egan's (2002) work and, similarly, has been criticized for being too prescriptive. However, where Egan's work is centered on problem management,

Page and Wosket (2001) focused on exploration and flexibility, appealing to a solution-focus.

Carroll's (1996) *Seven Generic Tasks* of supervision has been criticized for inflating the image of the supervisor as an expert, which invites a tangible power imbalance in the supervisory relationship. We aim for a more collaborative approach. In an idealistic setting, we remain a curious facilitator inviting a solution-focus. Practitioners are viewed in the role of expert and answer probing questions that require evidence. For example, when a practitioner tells us a client is benefiting from their sessions in the forest, we ask "How do you know?" (Ratner et al., 2012). A useful aspect of this approach is identifying the supervisor's role as a coach (see later in this chapter), or perhaps guide, to personal and professional development on the part of the practitioner, though some see this as outside the supervisor's role.

As with all things in this book, we recommend focusing on the model speaking your language around your practice, as this will lead to a more seamless implementation. Since it seems that there are as many ways to practice therapy outdoors as there are practitioners, this attention on an individual's way of working is essential. Discover what works for you in supervision and do more of it. It is perfectly normal to try out a supervisor, and if you find their approach is unhelpful, or contrary to the way you prefer to work, find another one.

Supervision versus Counseling

Supervision should never feel like counseling even given that practitioners might need to let off steam, which could be restorative, and there needs to be space and safety for this to happen (Towler, 2009). Supervisors are often counselors too and will most likely use their counseling skills during supervision. Egan (2002) described good counseling skills fundamental to any counseling or coaching process, which is informed by humanism and focused on listening, immediacy, empathic understanding, and so on. However, relying on counseling skills alone in a supervisory process is not enough. We identify this as a major criticism of the traditional person-centered approach (PCA). For Pearson (2006), boundaries are blurred when supervision feels like therapy, and ignores ethical issues around fitness to practice. Additionally, there may be insufficient structure to guide the supervisor in their role, who might, for example, avoid discussion issues relating to organizational policies and procedures that impact on the practitioner's work. Nonetheless, PCA has a significant role in our practice when giving and holding space for a fellow practitioner, just try not to confuse counseling with supervision.

Lambers (2007) argued person-centered practices facilitate experiences for cognitive and emotional learning or development. Exploring the supervisory relationship from the perspective of person-centered therapy, Villas-Boas Bowen (1986) found supervisors to trust the practitioner's inner resources and their capacity for self-direction. Allowing space for a practitioner to explore their work was examined by Casement (1985), who paid particular attention to the practitioner's voice and experience while supervising. Supervisors should communicate a non-judgmental and accepting stance, while treating all practitioners with unconditional positive regard, just as Rogerian counselors do. There follows a challenge to maintain acceptance and congruence with the practitioner, while continuing to work ethically in the best interest of co-adventurers and the field of outdoor therapy.

Our framework is flexible, with less rigid yet robust criteria. Context changes priorities in supervision (McLeod & Machin, 2008) in ways one could not fully predict. Borders (1989) has suggested methodical models of supervision suitable for working with novice practitioners. Supervisors should stay mindful, however, of the stage of a practitioner's development, as insufficient matching can lead to demoralization and stalled development. At the same time, one must be cautious of Hawkins and Shohet's (2009) warning that supervisors are not solely responsible for another's development, no more than solution-focused practitioners are for client change. Likewise, Borders (1989) argued that supervision, as we know it, maintains an insufficient emphasis on co-working and shared responsibility between the supervisor and the supervised. The focus tends to center on the supervisor, rather than on collaboration, trust, and the shared adventure that is impactful supervision.

Supervision versus Coaching

Most licensed therapists require supervision. It is probably a good thing, though the relationship between supervision and improved experiences for those we serve remains questionable (Watkins Jr., 2011). As we argued at the start of this chapter, if your supervisor cannot watch you work, they only rely on what you tell them about your therapeutic encounters. Including outcome and alliance data can help, though your supervisor will never be able to know what occurs when you are performing in front of your co-adventurer(s). We highly recommend getting a coach, perhaps in addition to supervision. This is an argument for perhaps having different supervisors who specialize in different aspects of your work. Find someone who will watch recordings of your work, examine your outcome data, and invest in strategies to develop areas requiring improvement. This is not recommending you read a landmark psychotherapy book or spend your weekend traveling to a workshop where you will learn a new technique cleverly marketed to radically help your clients in record time. While both could be fun, the evidence tells us neither will make you more effective (Chow et al., 2015). We need deliberate practice.

In outdoor therapy, a coach is someone invested in your development to improve service delivery and outcomes. They can schedule times for you to practice, maybe through role plays, or use recordings of your work to discuss areas in need of calibrating. If there is a practitioner you look up to, someone you wish you could emulate in your own work, get them on the phone and inquire about their coaching. Are they willing to watch you work? Are they equipped to discuss outcome and alliance data? This is an emerging area of our field and informs our work. We recommend reading Rousmaniere (2017), Miller et al. (2020), and Chow et al. (2015) for more information about deliberate practice.

A quick Google search of "deliberate practice rock climbing" will return lots of results, hence the relevance of Royal Robbins' (1994) quote to start the chapter. Page one of the results includes many articles about what climbers can do to improve their performance on the rock wall. Most of the relevant blog posts and articles stress that climbers wanting to advance require coaching. That coach should be someone who watches your work and develops a plan to improve your capabilities. Maybe you should work on strength training, finger strength, flexibility, or positioning on the wall. In essence, the coach helps to fine tune your skills, so you perform better when you are on the next route. Similarly, fine tuning your skills when you are away from your co-adventurers is important. Climbers seldom blame the rock wall for an unsuccessful climb, just as practitioners should avoid blaming clients for a lack of therapeutic progress. Therapy failures are opportunities for practitioners to up their skill. This only becomes possible when we humbly consider how we missed the mark or the areas of our therapeutic performance requiring deliberate practice. Practice does not make perfect. Practice makes better (Miller et al., 2020).

Supervisory Relationships

In many large agencies, a practitioner's clinical supervisor may also be their line manager. A danger associated with this is that a safe space to discuss a stuck case can quickly turn into an evaluation of job performance. We do not believe these two roles can be balanced, though they do require careful attention as they do get confused. Practitioners are more likely to report a benefit in supervision if they report a strong working relationship with their supervisor (Safran et al., 2008). These supervisors tend to put in the work, arrive prepared, and communicate genuine care for the practitioner's caseload and development.

Practitioners typically want to work on the issues they bring to supervision, such as mastering a specific skill, obtaining a better conceptualization of a stuck case, or working with a client beyond their perceived capabilities. Supervisors from varying theoretical perspectives may force an agenda of what they feel is most important, neglecting the practitioner's firsthand experience of working with these people. Supervisors should know about what practitioners do, though this may be asking a lot in the context of outdoor therapy. Still, if supervisors communicate they care about the practitioner's work, a relationship is nourished.

In our experience, supervisors should focus on engagement in supervision and the practitioner's view of the working relationship far beyond whatever model they choose. If the context of the supervision includes data from outcome monitoring, supervisors should take this process slow, as moving too fast could lead to a rupture in the relationship. Practitioners may feel cautious about sharing outcome data with someone they do not know well. This anxiety is heightened when the supervisor also maintains the role of line manager.

Supervisors are encouraged to ensure they are also informed by the best available evidence. This encourages a stance of humility when in the role of supervisor. We know some practitioners are more effective than others, and theoretical orientation or years of experience are no predictor one is more effective than the next (Chow et al., 2015). The supervisory relationship changes when supervisors acknowledge they may have no more privileged knowledge or increased effectiveness than the supervised, effectively taking a position of host leader. The supervisor is simply contracted to help practitioners make sense of their work and to focus the practitioner on developing to become more effective.

The following solution-focused questions are informed by the solution-focused practitioners at BRIEF in London and Bannink (2010). More questions are included in the manual in Appendix S.

- What will indicate you are getting what you want from supervision?
- What will tell me this supervision is beneficial for you?
- When we meet again next month, what would you tell me has been most useful?

- Have you experienced useful supervision in the past? If so, what did you find particularly useful?
- What should I know about your practice so I can best tailor the supervision?
- What will you/clients/managers/teachers notice that indicates this time in supervision is useful?
- If I recorded the way you work currently, and then again six months later, what would I notice?
- What do clients notice that is unique about your way of working?
- If I were to feel anxious about the way you were working with a particular case, how would you like us to handle that situation?
- What would your colleagues notice about your work that indicates supervision was useful?

Effective supervisors are able to describe their preferred method of supervision, no matter the type. We mentioned just a few informing our supervising and consultancy work and provided some relevant criticisms. While those models help us to track progress of the supervision, relationship trumps all. Any practitioner should feel cared for, held, and as though the supervisor is putting in the effort to understand the context of their work. This becomes difficult in outdoor therapies as the supervisor might practice comfortably from an office in the city. No matter their wealth of experience or knowledge, they should take time to understand the rationale for your work and believe in what you do. Their aim is to help you get better at doing it – not for you to be more like them.

Future research on the topic of deliberate practice is required in outdoor therapy. Most outdoor therapy practitioners obtain a qualification relevant to practice in their respective country, or state, and they are on their way. Training in outdoor therapy is limited and, at this stage, we have no data to suggest how to best train people to be effective in outdoor therapy. Thus, as you are sure to have noticed, we routinely borrow evidence from psychotherapy as a broad and diverse field to acknowledge the limitations of our current knowledge base and seek possibilities of solutions. Much of our work goes unobserved or without evaluation, the importance of asking questions about our practice not only relates to safety, it relates to the development of a field of practice we can unequivocally call evidence-informed, or evidence-based if you prefer. Like striving for excellence, these are not destinations, they are practices, a verb, an action that practitioners do to continue to get better each day.

Conclusion

Taking therapy outdoors requires careful consideration regarding supervision. We urge practitioners to use the data they build from client feedback to inform the supervision they receive. There are many models to consider and the alliance between supervisor and the supervised requires ongoing attention to prevent ruptures. Though supervision is important for ensuring client welfare, the direct correlation between supervision and enhanced outcomes for our co-adventurers is limited. Finding a coach who can observe your work and focus on locating areas requiring ongoing development is critical for improving your effectiveness, and a good supervisor would be able to do this for you. The following chapter brings this book to a close. We will link to ideas for advancing outdoor therapy's evidence base and provide some thoughts on striving for excellence.

References

Abiddin, N. Z. (2008). Exploring clinical supervision to facilitate the creative process of supervision. *Journal of International Sociology Research, 1*(3), 13–32.

Aten, J. D., Strain, J. D., & Gillespie, R. E. (2008). A transtheoretical model of clinical supervision. *Training and Education in Professional Psychology, 2*(1), 1–9. https://doi.org/10.1037/1931-3918.2.1.1

Bannink, F. (2010). *1001 solution-focused questions: Handbook for solution-focused interviewing.* W. W. Norton & Co.

Bargmann, S. (2017). *Achieving excellence through feedback-informed supervision.* In D. S. Prescott, C. L. Maeschalck, & S. D. Miller (Eds.), *Feedback-informed treatment in clinical practice: Reaching for excellence* (pp. 79–100). American Psychological Association. https://doi.org/10.1037/0000039-005

Borders, L. D. (1989). Developmental cognitions of first practicum supervisees. *Journal of Counseling Psychology, 36*(2), 163–169.

Caldwell, B. E. (2015). *Saving psychotherapy: How therapists can bring the talking cure back from the brink.* Ben Caldwell Labs.

Carroll, M. (1996). *Counselling supervision: Theory, skills, and practice.* Sage.

Casement, P. (2013). *Further learning from the patient: The analytic space and process.* Routledge.

Chow, D. L., Miller, S. D., Seidel, J. A., Kane, R. T., Thornton, J. A., & Andrews, W. P. (2015). The role of deliberate practice in the development of highly effective psychotherapists. *Psychotherapy, 52*(3), 337–345. https://doi.org/10.1037/pst0000015

Davys, A., & Beddoe, L. (2010). *Best practice in professional supervision: A guide for the helping professions.* Jessica Kingsley Publishing.

Dobud, W. W., & Cavanaugh, D. L. (2020). Future direction for outdoor therapies. In N. J. Harper & W. W. Dobud (Eds.), *Outdoor therapies: An introduction to practices, possibilities, and critical perspectives* (pp. 188–202). Routledge.

Egan, G. (2002). *The skilled helper* (7th ed.) Brooks/Cole.

Hawkins, P., & Schwenk, G. (2009). The interpersonal relationship in the training and supervision of coaches. In S. Palmer & A. McDowell (Eds.), *The coaching relationship: Putting people first.* Essential coaching skills and knowledge. Routledge.

Hawkins, P., & Shohet, R. (2009). *Supervision in the helping professions.* Open University Press.

Inskipp, F., & Proctor, B. (2001). *The art, craft, and tasks of counselling supervision: Part 2, Becoming a supervisor* (2nd ed.) Cascade Publications.

Kaberry, S. (2000). Abuse in supervision. In B. Lawton & C. Feltham (Eds.), *Taking supervision forward: Enquiries and trends in counselling and psychotherapy* (pp. 42–58). SAGE Publications.

Lambers, E. (2007). A person-centred perspective on supervision. In M. Cooper, M. O'Hara, P. F. Schmid, & G. Wyatt (Eds.), *The handbook of person-centred psychotherapy and counselling* (pp. 366–378). Palgrave Macmillan.

McLeod, J., & Machin, L. (1998). The context of counselling: A neglected dimension of training, research and practice. *British Journal of Guidance & Counselling,* 26(3), 325–336. https://doi.org/10.1080/03069889800760291

Miller, S. D., Hubble, M. A., & Chow, D. (2020). *Better results: Using deliberate practice to improve therapeutic effectiveness.* American Psychological Association.

Natynczuk, S., & Dobud, W. W. (2021). Leave no trace, willful unknowing, and implications from the ethics of sustainability for solution-focused practice outdoors. *Journal of Solution Focused Practices,* 5(2), 7.

Newnham-Kanas, C., Morrow, D., & Irwin, J. D. (2010). Motivational coaching: A functional juxtaposition of three methods for health behaviour change: Motivational interviewing, coaching, and skilled helping. *International Journal of Evidence Based Coaching and Mentoring,* 8(2), 27–48.

O'Donovan, A., Halford, W. K., & Walters, B. (2011). Towards best practice supervision of clinical psychology trainees. *Australian Psychologist, 46,* 101–112. https://doi.org/10.1111/j.1742-9544.2011.00033.x

Page, S., & Wosket, V. (2001). The cyclical model of supervision: A container for creativity and chaos. In M. Carroll & M. Tholstrup (Eds.), *Integrative approaches to supervision*. Jessica Kingsley Publishing.

Pearson, Q. M. (2006). Psychotherapy-driven supervision: Integrating counseling theories into role-based supervision. *Journal of Mental Health Counseling, 28*(3), 241–252. https://doi.org/10.17744/mehc.28.3.be1106w7yg3wvt1w

Ratner, H., George, E., & Iveson, C. (2012). *Solution focused brief therapy: 100 key points and techniques*. Routledge.

Robbins, R. (1994). *Basic rockcraft*. LA Siesta Pr.

Rousmaniere, T. (2017). *Deliberate practice for psychotherapists: A guide to improving clinical effectiveness*. Routledge.

Safran, J. D., Muran, J. C., Stevens, C., & Rothman, M. (2008). A relational approach to supervision: Addressing ruptures in the alliance. In C. A. Falender & E. P. Shafranske (Eds.), *Casebook for clinical supervision: A competency-based approach* (pp. 137–157). American Psychological Association. https://doi.org/10.1037/11792-007

Schwenk, E., & Natynczuk, S. (2015). Supervision and adventure therapy: Fighting burnout and providing emotional first aid for practitioners. In C. L. Norton, C. Carpenter, & A. Pryor (Eds.), *Adventure therapy around the globe: International perspectives and diverse approaches* (pp. 608–630). Common Ground.

Shulman, L. (2005). The clinical supervisor-practitioner working alliance: A parallel process. *The Clinical Supervisor, 24*(1–2), 23–47. https://doi.org/10.1300/J001v24n01_03

Towler, J. (2009). Friend or foe? The influence of the invisible client. *Counselling at Work*, 2–7.

Villas-Boas Bowen, M. C. (1986). Personality differences and person-centered supervision. *Person-Centered Review, 1*(3), 291–309.

Watkins, C. E., Jr. (2011). Does psychotherapy supervision contribute to patient outcomes? Considering thirty years of research. *The Clinical Supervisor, 30*(2), 235–256. https://doi.org/10.1080/07325223.2011.619417

Wosket, V. (2006). *Egan's skilled helper model: Developments and applications in counselling*. Routledge.

Žorga, S. (2007). Competencies of a supervisor. *Ljetopis socijalnog rada, 14* (2), 433–441.

11
Concluding Thoughts

"Steps to become a positive deviant: 1. Ask unscripted questions. 2. Don't complain. 3. Count something that interests you. 4. Write something... Anything. 5. Change yourself. Change something."

Atul Gawande (2008, pp. 249–257)

In this final chapter, we bring in some future considerations for outdoor therapy providers. We do provide some ideas for future research, though keep this brief as these ideas have been discussed previously and are highlighted throughout the book. We touch on the need for us to take a stand in relation to ethics and holding ourselves and peers accountable to best practice. We conclude this book with a discussion on how you can bring a *culture of excellence* into your practice, aiming to improve outdoor therapy outcomes one co-adventurer, one adventure at a time.

We are fond of Dr. Atul Gawande's work, staff writer for the *New Yorker*, and author of many books relating to surgical safety and improving medical outcomes. We cannot recommend reading his works enough. The quote above comes from his book *Better: A Surgeon's Notes on Performance* (2008). As we go through this final chapter, we examine outdoor therapies through the lens of positive deviance. This idea for behavioral change came from researchers inquiring into the behavior of the most well-nourished children in impoverished communities, despite social determinants and risk factors. The researchers created a program based on what these outlier families were doing. Malnutrition fell by 85%. Results were sustained.

Applying positive deviance to outdoor therapies is important. If the field continues as is, there will be people doing great, yet overwhelmingly unnoticed work. Historically, outdoor therapy providers did something very brave. They opened the counseling room door and shared the great outdoors with those who sought their help. They asked questions about how this all

DOI: 10.4324/9781003217558-14

works and began building evidence using similar methodologies to psychotherapy's big hitters. They chronicled their work in peer-reviewed papers and books and advocated for third party reimbursement or more funding from local governments. Unfortunately, those have been the actions of the few.

Even without a background in conducting research, we encourage all of you to become scientists of the world, and your practice. Ask questions about what is working, ask your co-adventurers what makes your practice effective, and write about it. Our field has an old and rusted dominant narrative with aspects of unethical, unsafe, and punitive practices. We need to deviate from this in order to construct a richer narrative about outdoor therapies. We need to learn from the outliers in our field. What do the most impactful do differently? What are the keys to their successes? What do their clients say about them? Asking these big picture questions can help us to build awareness that outdoor therapies are not just for the few. They are being practiced all over the world. To gain a rightful seat at the psychotherapy table, we have to build evidence – qualitatively, quantitatively – in any way possible.

Future Research

Further integrating adventure, leadership, talking, and experiential therapies to enhance therapeutic relationships requires ongoing research to know what is effective for those coming to therapy. Adding to this, we are up against the cognitive-behavioral tsunami (Dalal, 2018), influenced by neoliberalism, managerialist ideologies, and unjustified overinflation of efficacy. The privileging of specific research methodologies, namely randomized clinical trials, has led to perceiving outdoor therapies as lesser than to those with greater evidence bases. Of course, we need to build evidence, and feedback-informed treatment is one way to not only improve our clients' experiences but build reliable outcome data. Just make sure you do not simply use the measures for evaluating your work: that is not their sole, intended purpose. Clients' voices are essential to hear. These methods are designed solely to improve client experiences.

The Streetlight Effect

What many practitioners do outdoors works. Outdoor therapy outcomes remain on par with those from tightly controlled clinical trials. We are not divided only by how we refer to our work, such as nature-based or wilderness therapy, but also by the theoretical frameworks informing our perspective.

Thus, a cognitive-behavioral counselor and a psychoanalytic psychiatrist may both refer to their work as adventure therapy, yet how they conceptualize their work is drastically different. Simply researching wilderness therapy programs with the assumption that we know what effects we are observing seems to miss the point. We fear outdoor therapies have fallen into the trap of using simple-to-ask questions to inform our research agendas. This, as many of you know, leads to what is called the *streetlight effect*.

Imagine you leave a restaurant on a busy and cold Friday night. Under the streetlight, a drunk is looking in the light for his wallet. You ask him where he thinks he last saw it and he points off into the dark and foggy distance. He is only looking under the streetlight because the light is better there. This seems to be how most psychotherapy research is conducted. We tend to ask the easiest questions we can at the expense of being rigorous. There is no doubt our outcome data is robust and growing, yet we can follow clues from other psychotherapy research to learn more about outdoor therapy encounters.

When digesting outcome research, we should ask an important question. Does this research show that therapeutic initiatives, in general, work? Or does it show there are some unique factors about this approach that contribute to outcomes? For example, proponents of outdoor behavioral healthcare have spent the better part of two decades conceptualizing how wilderness therapy works. Their papers include arguments that the social milieu, therapist's role, time in nature, specific outdoor activities, and family involvement are the ingredients contributing to outcome (e.g., Gass et al., 2019). Without a comparison group omitting these factors, it is a hard sell to suggest outdoor activities contribute anything to outcome. In fact, Dobud and Harper (2018) found that in the limited comparison groups where outdoor therapy was compared to anything even slightly different, with equivalent doses of treatment, no distinguishable difference in outcomes could be found.

This sounds damning. We assure you it is not. It is liberating. If we follow the available evidence, we know what practitioners do on average is effective. The setting where therapy takes place has no bearing on outcomes but provides yet another avenue to help those who seek our counsel. Research exists to show time outdoors can improve wellbeing. That does not equate to psychotherapy settings. We need to increase our evidence base to improve accessibility. Cognitive-behavioral therapy on a psychotherapist's couch should be just as accessible as an outdoor therapy expedition. We should not think we are more special than anything else, just different, and some people prefer to be outdoors.

We are not ignorant to the game outdoor therapy researchers must play to gain recognition as an empirically supported treatment. We must demonstrate our cost-effectiveness, outcomes, and safety. Advocates and practitioners should do everything they can to use their evidence to advocate for the potential of taking therapy out of the counseling room. The zoomed out and historical view of therapy outcomes, however, informs us that what we are likely to find is we are just as effective as anything else. No better, no worse. The therapy itself, whether solution-focused as we described in this book, will not always make the difference. Neither will nature. All of those things *could* work yet homogenizing all your co-adventurers to fit into your preferred model neglects the wild cards of therapy outcomes: the people involved. Instead of repeating tired pre-/post-outcome research focused on entire treatment protocols, Miller et al. (2010) argued we turn our attention "to the moment-by-moment, encounter-to-encounter processes associated with effective psychotherapy. Once identified, tested, and confirmed, the field is set to empower the next generation of therapists to emulate empirically derived patterns of excellence" (p. 425).

We simply do not have this data in relation to therapy outdoors, though many have tried. Russell and Gillis (2017) did important work with the development of the Adventure Therapy Experience Scale. However, uptake has been slow, much like our push for outcome monitoring. If you are not certain about what measures to use, you can certainly use Russell and Gillis' scale, along with an outcome measure, such as the ORS, to build data about moment-to-moment encounters. This will help researchers examine dose effect, being how long most people should spend in outdoor therapy settings to predict a positive response. Without this data, we will continue to make erroneous assumptions about whether therapy should be brief or long term. We will send young people to ongoing residential treatment when the outcomes are telling us they should return to their families and communities (Harper et al., 2021).

If we continue trekking along with our similar research agendas, we will continue to show that taking therapy outdoors can be effective for many, a just cause. We are unlikely, however, to improve our outcomes, a similar pitfall to the 1,000 or so modalities of psychotherapy (Miller et al., 2020). Instead of looking at the treatment itself, which makes up the feeblest share of <1% of variance in therapy outcomes, we need to look at what we know matters. This, we argue, can help us to improve our performance and achieve better results.

Adventure Therapy Outcome Monitoring (ATOM) Database

In 1974, a study was conducted by D. F. Ricks to explore a group of exceptional practitioners, who he referred to as *supershrinks*. He examined the longitudinal outcomes for highly disturbed teenagers. When those teens were adults, Ricks found that one group lived much more well-adjusted lives. The other group were remarkably worse off. The difference was the practitioner who worked with the young people. Despite this landmark finding, it has taken the better part of half a century to wake up to the fact that who delivers the therapeutic service is vastly more important than definitions, treatment protocols, manuals, diagnoses, or biopsychosocial assessments (Miller et al., 2020).

Along with colleagues, such as Dr. Daniel L. Cavanaugh in the United States, we have been working to establish the Adventure Therapy Outcome Monitoring (ATOM) Database. At this stage, the dataset has undergone a few revisions after consultation from leading psychotherapy researchers and has been resubmitted to an ethics committee for final approval. The ATOM database will invite practitioners from around the world to input their individual outcomes and style of their work to participate in what we intend to be the largest and most rigorous study of outdoor therapy. We discuss below the potential for this work. Watch this space.

We must take the variance in practitioner's outcomes seriously. The more practitioners we get to invest in outcome monitoring, the bigger database we can build to first argue that, yes, despite our diversity and heterogeneity in theoretical orientation, what we do as a collective works. Some, of course, are better than others, though establishing a research agenda focused on individual practitioners pays credence to what contributes most to the variance in outcomes. If this research grows as we intend, we can begin to learn from those eliciting the best outcomes.

There is little known about how outdoor therapy practitioners are trained or how they develop over their careers. With more practitioners establishing their baseline of effectiveness, researchers can begin piloting professional development packages to improve people's outcomes. By using outcome monitoring in this way, supervision and deliberate practice become evidence-based. The ATOM will hold clues as to what practitioners can do to get better. We can look at variances across professions, years of experience, outdoor setting, theoretical orientation, and so on. We hope you will participate with us. Everyone is welcome. To prepare for launch, we recommend implementing outcome monitoring with new co-adventurers.

At the start of this book, we argued that definitions of what is or is not a specific type of therapy is of little interest to us. Of course, this may be ironic given the theme and focus of this very book. Gass et al.'s (2020) definition asserts that adventure therapy must be delivered by mental health professionals. This is just one of many definitions of an outdoor therapy practitioner. We have close colleagues who have sought our supervision to make sense of their initial outcome data. One a police officer, another a youth worker and outdoor educator. Their work has elicited outcomes far above the averages for psychotherapy in general (Wampold & Imel, 2015)! What if they were the outdoor supershrinks? Our third party payers and insurance companies should want to know. Additionally, how amazing would it be to record and observe their work?

Predictors of Progress

When we build an inclusive database of individual practitioner outcomes, no matter the qualification, country of origin, gender identity, age, cultural background, years of experience, theoretical orientation, or any other identifiable factor, we can begin to seriously examine predictors of progress. If, like other critical research (e.g. Chow et al., 2015), we find the variables we listed above will not account for client change, what do we look for? What we should find are clues as to why some practitioners are able to facilitate more meaningful and engaging outdoor therapy experiences. The data we can develop using outcome and alliance measures will provide hints as to what patterns we should look out for, such as a low alliance measure after the first few days of an expedition.

Historically, we have examined therapeutic encounters based on variables we assume are most important. When this occurs, co-adventurers' experiences are silenced. We risk neglecting the co-adventurers' preferences and motivation. Many of those we work with do not arrive to our programs trauma-informed or solution-focused, or thinking they need more time in nature. They can do that themselves and probably do not need to pay for it. In fact, most of the time when people disengage from our services, it has nothing to do with what type of work we delivered. They do not leave and say, "You know, despite getting nothing from that session, I've got to hand it to Will and Stephan, at least they were evidence-based and outside." Most people disengage due to issues in the therapeutic relationship or a lack of progress early on (Miller et al., 2020).

We must abandon the assumptions we make about how we conceptualize outdoor therapy encounters. Time in nature *may* be healing, though it is the client who must feel that. Simply pushing our outdoor hobbies onto our clients is not enough to bring this wonderful field forward (Rosen, 2020). When we acknowledge that the interventions we use, whether sitting on a park bench or scaling a multi-pitch climb, have no inherent value, we are more open to finding what solution is best tailored to our client. We are awarded further humility when we realize that we have to *make these things work*. Interventions have no therapeutic value on their own. Where one co-adventurer may find sleeping under the stars peaceful and reflective, another feels homesick, scared, and falls into an existential crisis about their place in the universe. Context is everything. We know, inherently, it is all about how this work is *experienced* and the *meaning constructed*, which starts with how we describe the rationale of the work to our co-adventurers.

You may notice that our tone has shifted as we conclude this book. We admit, there is a bit of finger wagging and the old "Get off my lawn!" stereotype going on here. As we wrap this up, we want to assure you that the work and literature of others, including what we have written, are writing, and will continue to write, impacts all of us. When we talk about outdoor therapies, we are often asked about the worst and most unethical aspects that have occurred or critiqued about the limits of our evidence base. We are left defending a field, based on the actions of the few, instead of the promise of sharing the great outdoors with more wonderful people. We conclude here with the need to take a stand in the pursuit of excellence.

Taking a Stand

As well as our credentials as outdoor leaders, we hold degrees in social work, behavioral science, teaching, business, supervision, and counseling. These certificates gain us admittance to a select group of helping practitioners operating under one *professional umbrella*, such as the Australian Association of Social Workers, the National Counselling Society, or the British Association for Counselling and Psychotherapy. Throughout the book, we stressed that we do not privilege one type of training or practitioner over the next, but here we make a distinction about well-informed and ethical practice. We began this book with a call to action for practitioners to present the theories and techniques they use in their outdoor practice. To be considered a bona-fide psychotherapy, all models require a psychological rationale for how their service is effective and how the rituals they use link to that rationale (Frank & Frank, 1991; Wampold & Imel, 2015). With this book, we have presented one. Harper et al. (2019) presented another.

Collectively, the two of us have provided consultation for outdoor therapy providers in over 20 countries and have been in the field for a combined 50 years or more. There are times practitioners describe their work as holistic or integrative; words that communicate little about what they actually do (Caldwell, 2015). While many of us are passionate about being outside, this is not enough to become an outdoor therapy provider. We need training, a theoretical orientation, and a practice framework, including ethics, to justify our work. We must be able to define what we do pragmatically. Only then will we know if what we are doing is off-track or unethical.

We have heard: *If you think and don't do, you are useless. If you do and don't think, you are dangerous, or reckless.* Unfortunately, our experience has been that despite so many wonderfully passionate people working in this field, we have seen times when both of these statements are true.

In the states, it seems that some practitioners are compliant to the process of kidnapping youth to send them to wilderness therapy provision without the participant's consent in a process known as *transporting*. Accounts of this are given in books such as that by Kenneth Rosen (2020) and collected in my (Will's) doctoral thesis (2020, later published in 2021). Along with Nevin Harper and Doug Magnuson (2021), we questioned the ethics of such practice against social workers' ethics and the United Nations' (2017) *Mental Health and Human Rights* report. Views of what is in a client's best interests are thus hugely variable and acceptance of what is appropriate is definitely not the same across the world. The authors recall the amazement and horror from some international representatives that transporting was at all possible, while some sought to justify this practice. Thus, the diversity of what is acceptable makes a common ethics challenging to put it mildly.

When one graduates with their qualification, such as in social work or counseling, they join a unique professional club. When we begin practicing outdoors, our professional identity may shift from *social worker* to *outdoor therapist*. If we lose our identity as social workers, psychologists, youth workers, teachers, or whatever our profession, we may become complicit in practices at odds with our professional code of ethics. For example, many of the programs transporting adolescents to US wilderness therapy programs are delivered by licensed clinical social workers. In our advocacy work, we encourage them to revisit their duty as social workers first, outdoor practitioners second. The same goes for psychologists, counselors, and educators. We, the authors, are unashamedly against any provision of therapy that comes through deception, coercion, or is indistinguishable from punitive treatment. It is unethical.

Caldwell's (2015) brief and fantastic book, *Saving Psychotherapy: How Therapists Can Bring the Talking Cure Back from Brink,* encourages practitioners to "Take It Personally." We link to his arguments in providing some ideas on what we can collectively do to help our field grow and flourish.

The dangerous, unethical, or unsafe actions of other practitioners are a reflection on not only psychotherapy in general, but our close-knit outdoor therapy community. Our values must be made clear to prospective funders and co-adventurers. If we see unethical practice, we can call it out with kindness and offer to help. Never have we used a program or practitioner's name when striving for safer, more ethical programs. We hope they listen and make the necessary changes, and we are a phone call away from offering our consultation.

We must fight for those behind us. Gatekeeping practices keep many who have wonderful ideas, such as the police officer described previously, from feeling welcomed and necessary in moving our field forward. When asked how someone can get involved in this work, we discuss the many pathways and encourage people to let their passion and finances inform their decision. Once aspirant practitioners enter the field, we should provide supervision at reasonable costs and supervise students undergoing their required field placements.

Become an evidence-informed practitioner. Build evidence of your outcomes and client experiences and use data as a map to inform your decision making. Be a curious skeptic of research, not a cynic. We should be able to differentiate bad science from the good and understand the null hypothesis. Share your outcomes and please, *write* about your work. The narrative of outdoor therapies is dominated by the few, and the work you do is valid for publication. If you have something you want reviewed or edited, or just want plain consultation, we are willing to help. Your voice and evidence matters!

Publish the data you build each year, even if just on your website. What percentage of your co-adventurers achieved significantly reliable change? How long did it take them to do so? Your consumers and funders might want to know. Making your data public and transparent is key. Hold your colleagues, coworkers, and peers to a high standard. Practice the skill of gentle and compassionate confrontation. We are a caring profession, and it will typically only take a simple yet kind conversation to remind your peers about their ethical obligations.

Caldwell (2015) concludes with a call for us to become *activist therapists*. We want our work to be taken seriously, but many of us do not address the legalized kidnapping occurring every day under the guise of wilderness therapy. We must "protest that which is not working in our profession, and loudly champion what is" (p. 182). Shennan (2020) encouraged us to consider the possibilities of changing one word of our favorite question: "What are *our* best hopes as a community of outdoor therapy practitioners?" Being a therapist in your community is a position of leadership. We have an obligation to pursue required changes, even more so when others may not be ready.

We end here with Caldwell's (2015) final call to arms:

> Our profession is slowly eroding, doing particular harm to new professionals. It is hard to say how long this erosion will continue, how long we as a collective group might remain lost in the proverbial woods. You can lead us out. I hope and expect that if you take the actions outlined here, others will follow you. But if they do not, you can be one of those left standing.
> First, you have to stand.
>
> (pp. 182–183)

Striving for Excellence

In 2018, I (Will) participated in the first delivery of psychologist Dr. Daryl Chow's (2021) course *Reigniting Clinical Supervision*. While my organization had already successfully implemented routine outcome monitoring, I was still developing as a supervisor for social work and outdoor therapy practice. The course, which we highly recommend, provided a new strategy for how we manage the small team of practitioners and students we work with. This framework is informed by groundwork we have presented in Chapters 2, 9, and 10. We recommend implementing this in your agency, and have never looked back ourselves.

On Monday morning, our team meets around a table with coffee and maybe some breakfast. A different person each week will review our mission as outdoor therapy practitioners. What this does not mean is reading some mission statement written years ago, remaining buried on the company's website. We want it to come from the heart; to inspire us for the week. Think about your values and write them down. Use them to motivate you to be the best worker you can be. Based on that mission, each of us writes, using the same template in Appendix T, what we will measurably do to achieve this ambition. Keep it brief. A sentence or two. Nothing too big. It might be to return phone calls at a faster rate or to send some additional resources to a parent to remind them you have got their back. Avoid being overly theoretical, stay task focused for this. The thing about mission statements that many people overlook is that they must be measurable: that is how we know we are developing our practice.

In the afternoon, Friday, we meet again around the same table before breaking for the weekend. This meeting tends to be filled with laughter, which helps cushion the vulnerability. When new workers join our team, we are excited by the look they give us when they experience this ritual; especially our interns who just wanted to work therapeutically outdoors. The purpose of this meeting is to *capture our weekly learnings*. Said another way, think about the areas of our work in need of attention and improvement. Maybe you received a bad session rating or did not review your case notes thoroughly enough before a subsequent session. Capture a little thing that went wrong. You do not want to forget it.

Everyone participates: the clinical director, the outdoor guides, the licensed psychotherapist, and the students on placement. It is vital for those in positions of power to model a culture of feedback and excellence. We all know mistakes happen, and we are not immune by nailing diplomas and various pieces of paper to the wall. We have to capture these little issues so we can address them. The following Monday, your action for the week should address the weekly learning you captured on Friday. This goes on each and every week.

If you are disciplined enough to do this for one year, you will end up with at least 52 things you have learned, and the specific actions you set for yourself to improve your work. Remember, our theories, qualifications, or the number of expensive weekend workshops we attend do not correlate with improved individual outcomes (Miller et al., 2020). Neither does the number of clients we have worked with previously, if we are indoors or out, or the years we have spent providing clinical psychotherapy (Dobud & Harper, 2018; Chow et al., 2015). We have to focus on *getting better* at whatever it is we do. While we discussed core competencies in Chapter 8, the road to excellence is much more challenging. Add the outdoors and the necessary qualifications for demonstrating said competence, and it becomes further muddied.

Conclusion (At the Time of Writing)

Solution-focused therapy outdoors is nothing new (Gass & Gillis, 1995), though the framework has required further examination and unpacking. We have maintained that while we need a model, like solution-focused, to inform our outdoor work, we must take seriously what certain models contribute to our effectiveness as a field. To do this, we have provided strategies and ideas for building your own evidence and taking a stand to make outdoor therapy sustainable, ethical, and accessible.

What we have presented is how us two have worked for over half a century. There are other ways to conceptualize and deliver therapy outdoors effectively. We love the diversity of outdoor therapies and by no means wish to homogenize it. We know of trauma-informed professionals doing amazing work and the field of psychotherapy really beginning to explore the impact of trauma is vastly important. The literature on the topic, in relation to outdoor therapies, however, is missing. We hope books like this one, and those that will follow, help practitioners to know what to do and when to do it, how to think about their co-adventurers, and improve all of our abilities to make evidence-informed decisions when stuck in the thick of it.

Stay safe and happy co-adventuring!

References

Caldwell, B. E. (2015). *Saving psychotherapy: How therapists can bring the talking cure back from the brink*. Ben Caldwell Labs.

Chow, D. L. (2018). Re-igniting clinical supervision: Taking clinical supervisors and psychotherapists to next level of real development. Retrieved from https://darylchowcourses.teachable.com/p/reignitingsupervision

Chow, D. L., Miller, S. D., Seidel, J. A., Kane, R. T., Thornton, J. A., & Andrews, W. P. (2015). The role of deliberate practice in the development of highly effective psychotherapists. *Psychotherapy*, 52(3), 337–345. https://doi.org/10.1037/pst0000015

Dalal, F. (2018). *CBT: The cognitive behavioural tsunami: Managerialism, politics and the corruptions of science*. Routledge.

Dobud, W. W. (2020). *Experiences of adventure therapy: A narrative inquiry* [Doctoral Dissertation]. Charles Sturt University.

Dobud, W. W., & Harper, N. J. (2018). Of dodo birds and common factors: A scoping review of direct comparison trials in adventure therapy. *Complementary Therapies in Clinical Practice*, 31, 16–24. https://doi.org/10.1016/j.ctcp.2018.01.005

Frank, J. D., & Frank, J. B. (1991). *Persuasion and healing: A comparative study of psychotherapy*. JHU Press.

Gass, M. A., & Gillis, H. L. (1995). Focusing on the "solution" rather than the "problem": Empowering client change in adventure experiences. *Journal of Experiential Education*, 18(2), 63–69. https://doi.org/10.1177%2F105382599501800202

Gass, M. A., Gillis, H. L., & Russell, K. C. (2020). *Adventure therapy: Theory, research, and practice* (2nd ed.) Routledge.

Gass, M. A., Wilson, T., Talbot, B., Tucker, A., Ugianskis, M., & Brennan, N. (2019). The value of outdoor behavioral healthcare for adolescent substance users with comorbid conditions. *Substance Abuse: Research and Treatment, 13*. https://doi.org/10.1177/1178221819870768

Gawande, A. (2008). Better: A surgeon's notes on performance. Profile Books.

Harper, N. J., Magnuson, D., & Dobud, W. W. (2021). A closer look at involuntary treatment and the use of transport service in outdoor behavioral healthcare (wilderness therapy). *Child & Youth Services, 42*(2), 1–20. https://doi.org/10.1080/0145935X.2021.1938526

Harper, N. J., Rose, K., & Segal, D. (2019). *Nature-based therapy: A practitioner's guide to working outdoors with children, youth, and families.* New Society Publishers.

Miller, S. D., Hubble, M. A., & Chow, D. (2020). *Better results: Using deliberate practice to improve therapeutic effectiveness.* American Psychological Association.

Miller, S. D., Hubble, M. A., Duncan, B. L., & Wampold, B. E. (2010). Delivering what works. In B. L. Duncan, S. D. Miller, B. E. Wampold, & M. A. Hubble (Eds.), *The heart and soul of change: Delivering what works in therapy* (2nd ed.) (pp. 421–429). American Psychological Association.

Ricks, D. F. (1974). Supershrink: Methods of a therapist judged successful on the basis of adult outcomes of adolescent patients. In D. F. Ricks, A. Thomas, & M. Roff (Eds.), *Life history research in psychopathology* (Vol. 3). University of Minnesota Press.

Rosen, K. (2020). *Troubled: The failed promise of America's behavioral programs.* Little A.

Russell, K., & Gillis, H. L. (2017). The adventure therapy experience scale: The psychometric properties of a scale to measure the unique factors moderating an adventure therapy experience. *Journal of Experiential Education, 40*(2), 135–152. https://doi.org/10.1177%2F1053825917690541

Shennan, G. (2020). Towards a critical solution-focused practice? *Journal of Solution Focused Practices, 4*(1), 15–21.

United Nations. (2017). *Mental health and human rights: Report of the United Nations high commissioner for human rights.* Annual report of the United Nations High Commissioner for Human Rights and reports of the Office of the High Commissioner and the Secretary General. Retrieved from www.un.org/disabilities/documents/reports/ohchr/a_hrc_34_32_mental_health_and_human_rights_2017.docx

Wampold, B. E., & Imel, Z. E. (2015). *The great psychotherapy debate: The evidence for what makes psychotherapy work* (2nd ed.) Routledge.

Appendix
Field Manual for Solution-Focused Practice Outdoors

Appendix A – Outdoor Solution-Focused Field Manual

Imagine a moment on a training course for outdoor instructors, half a dozen people huddled in a cave discussing emergency rope-work and the usefulness of having an additional karabiner or "krab." An obvious visual and word pun causes some amusement, a few groans. *Spare Krab* is born.

That was possibly well over 15 years and many adventures ago. Zoom forwards through time, colleagues and former students regularly ask, often with genuine affection: "How's *Spare Krab* doing?" "What adventures have there been since we last met?"

Back in 2019, at an adventure therapy conference, I (Stephan) sat with a small group of friends on a veranda, Bavarian Alps framing the sunset, beer in hand. They teased, we laughed, then the banter became serious as a strong suggestion came. "*Spare Krab* is a good brand, and you should go with it!"

We talked about the long back story, the many anecdotes. "It's such an easily remembered name, an obvious logo, an amusing icon for serious training yet with a sense of fun. It's you Stephan." The enthusiasm was infectious.

Quickly checking something on his phone another participant announced, "If you're into this – an aligned spirit totem animal for whom not all paths lead directly to personal goals, a sideways approach being necessary. The crab spirit is protective of oneself yet recognizes community as vital to growth, introspective seclusion is important for growth and development. It is crucial to nourish your curiosity on all levels – the exploration of the wider world leading to new horizons and a vibrant life."

It was perfect.

spare krab

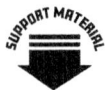

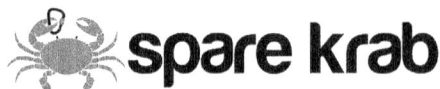

Figure A.1 Spare Krab logo

Our field manual was produced with you in mind. It is designed to be printed and laminated for your next therapeutic adventure. Each section of the manual is signposted throughout the book when described. We hope you find it useful as these checklists, worksheets, and tables help you to maintain a solution-focus in your outdoor therapy work.

Spare Krab is a great metaphor for growing, shedding the old confines, ecdysis. A moment of vulnerability as the soft new shell hardens before moving on, better equipped, bigger, stronger, refreshed to explore once again. It all seems to fit. There's certainly a helpful alignment with our core interest in outdoor and adventure therapy, with something new and vibrant about it. So, there we are: *Spare Krab*!

Please feel free to share a picture of this book or field manual on your next adventure, whether reading next to a campfire or while enjoying a sunset at the beach. Use #CoAdventuring, #OutdoorTherapy, or #SpareKrab so we can find you!

Happy and safe adventuring,

Will and Stephan

Outline

SUPPORT MATERIAL

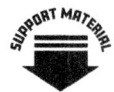

Appendix O – Interpreting Outcomes and Alliance Measures
Appendix P – Progress Report
Appendix Q – Feedback-Informed Supervision Table
Appendix R – Format for Evidence-Informed Supervision Outdoors
Appendix S – Questions for Solution-Focused Supervision
Appendix T – Striving for Excellence

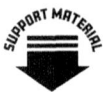

Appendix B – Tenets of Solution-Focused Practice

What We Think about Clients

- Every person is unique.
- People come to us with resources and strengths, both personal and in their social networks.
- All clients have the ability to find their own solutions to the difficulties they have.
- One cannot change clients; they can only change themselves.
- The therapy practitioner is not the expert on the client or their social network; the client is.
- A client's own solution that fits their own situation is more likely to be implemented and maintained than something suggested to them.

What We Think about Problems

- No problem happens all the time: there are always exceptions that can be found and built upon.
- A focus on the possible and changeable is more helpful than a focus on the overwhelming and intractable.
- The client is not the problem. The problem is the problem.
- The problem and the solution occur in the interaction between people rather than residing within people.
- Problems that appear complex might not require a complex solution.

What We Think about Change

- Change is constant.
- Small changes can make a big difference.
- Rapid change or resolution can happen when people hit on ideas that work.
- Change is likely to occur sooner rather than later.
- There may have been some pre-session change.

What We Think about Practice

- Lasting change is more likely to happen when you find out what is working and help people focus on what happens when they do more of it.
- Change is happening all the time. Our job is to identify and amplify useful change.
- People are more likely to behave and/or think differently when you work with their ideas of useful change.

Appendix C – Language Games

The use of language is critical to solution-focused practice. Not just in a deep philosophical Wittgensteinian way, in an everyday practical way. Care is taken about the use of words and the meaning they convey. We cannot assume clients understand the meaning we prescribe to the words we use. Examples of everyday words that can be less than useful in our solution-focused practice are presented in the table below.

Table A.1 Language Games in Outdoor Solution-Focused Practice

Words	Considerations for Outdoor Therapy Practice
But	Everything that comes after "but" stinks. This word negates what comes before it and can be experienced as dismissive. "I hear what you say but…" and "Yes, but…" are not helpful and sound like an argument rather than validating another's experience. Use other sentence connectors like "yet," "though," and "and" to signal acknowledgement of what you are hearing and to build on it.
Why?	This word can be experienced as requiring a justification and can be heard as judgmental. Practitioners are encouraged to avoid asking questions beginning with "why" and instead ask "how" participants were able to successfully implement change, instead of why they did or did not. Even better, ask what they noticed when the change occurred.
Do	Avoid language associated with tasks and lists. Concentrate on the signs of change. The tasks will seem to sort themselves out. Try it.
Diagnosis	As stated before, the mushrooming of diagnoses has not provided relief to ongoing mental health crises. For solution-focused practitioners, it is not our role to work out what is "wrong" with a client. Additionally, in the spirit of privileging self-determination and agency, we avoid trying to solve people's problems for them as this mimics the colonization of vulnerable people, and is quite paternalistic (Natynczuk & Dobud, 2021).

(Continued)

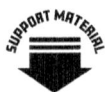

Table A.1 Language Games in Outdoor Solution-Focused Practice (*Cont'd*)

Words	Considerations for Outdoor Therapy Practice
Should *Ought* *Must*	We avoid "shoulding" on people. It is not our role to tell a client what to do unless it relates to physical safety. If we prescribe solutions to our co-adventurers, we risk becoming solution-forced and creating ruptures to the therapeutic alliance. Working on anything other than a person's best hopes is likely to increase disengagement and risk dropout.
When I was *If I were you*	Clients may ask for advice and care is required when responding. If our advice proves useful, your client may increase hope and expectancy that you are the right person to work with. The contrary, however, will reduce hope in the therapy alleviating their distress. In our ever progressing aim to decenter the therapist from the encounter, appropriating what has worked for you onto another person who has their own strengths, capabilities, resources, and exceptions is unadvised.
Stop	We would not ask "What is stopping you from doing…?" as this is too close to problem-focused talk. We are not interested in analyzing obstacles to progress, more about what the client would notice once any obstacle has been handled or overcome, like a stream moving around, under, or over a rock.

Language considerations are important. Because solution-focused practitioners resist the natural urge to be an expert in someone else's lived experience, it is important to reflect on words capable of demoralizing the participant. Instead, we view ourselves as a practitioner with some technical knowledge about outdoor pursuits and use our carefully crafted questions to gently guide co-adventurers to a more hopeful future.

Appendix D – The Crucial C's

When reflecting on a client's experience, you can use this template for guiding you to consider how your client is experiencing the *Crucial C's* we have adapted from the work of Lew and Bettern (1996).

Table A.2 Utilizing the Crucial C's in Outdoor Therapy Practice

What is the co-adventurer's experience of **connection**?
Does the co-adventurer feel they have **capability** to participate fully in your work?
Does the co-adventurer feel as though they **count** and that they can make a difference in your work?
Has the co-adventurer experienced opportunities to have **courage**?

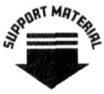

Appendix E – Am I Being Solution-Forced?

Table A.3 Solution-Forced Reflection for Outdoor Therapy Practitioners

Have I acknowledged and validated the client's experience of the problem?
Am I delivering the service or asking questions in a mechanical or instrumental manner? Is the client experiencing an "authentic" relationship?
Am I searching or advocating for exceptions/solutions that make no difference to the client?
Am I pushing for what I think is most important, and disregarding the client's preferred future?
Have I constructed a therapeutic climate of respect, curiosity, transparency, and openness?

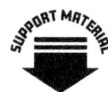

Appendix F – Host Leadership Roles in Outdoor Therapy

Table A.4 Reflection on Host Leadership Roles in Outdoor Therapy

	Role	Considerations for My Practice				
In Preparation	Initiator	My strengths in this area: Areas in need of development:				
	Inviter	My strengths in this area: Areas in need of development:				
	Space Creator	My strengths in this area: Areas in need of development:				
During the Experience	Gatekeeper	My strengths in this area: Areas in need of development:				
	Connector	My strengths in this area: Areas in need of development:				
	Co-Participator	My strengths in this area: Areas in need of development:				

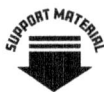

Appendix G – Leave No Trace Ethics in Outdoor Therapy Practice

For a full description of how Leave No Trace sustainability ethics can inform outdoor solution-focused practice see Natynczuk and Dobud (2021).

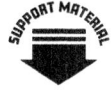

Table A.5 Principles of Leave No Trace for Solution-Focused Outdoor Therapy

Leave No Trace	Outdoor Practice	General Therapeutic Practice	Solution-Focused Practice
Plan Ahead and Prepare	• Consent and contracting. • Appropriate medical history. • Thorough risk assessment is recommended. • Choice of venue, route, timings, duration, location of facilities, pacing, late return/ emergency call-out and communication, local byelaws, access, maps, compass, technical equipment, clothing with regard to climate and weather forecast, spare clothing, head torches, first aid kit, emergency shelter, facility to make a hot drink and so forth.	• Being able to cope with unexpected occurrences takes on a new meaning, especially in unfamiliar environments. • Walk and talk pace can be very slow, the weather has a huge impact. • Terrain has to be appropriate to clients' fitness – it is difficult to talk when out of breath. • Pacing conversation with respect to the effort of moving. • Know places on your route where privacy is easier to find. • For short walks know the route, timings and places you can stand aside from the path while deep contemplation occurs. • There are so many metaphors in the outdoors that can help or hinder. • Understand the importance of landscape and how environment and nature can interact as co-facilitator. • Anticipate the impact of distractions, such as playful dogs and chatty interlopers. • Know how to finish the session if the route outlasts the conversation or vice versa.	• Clients bring their own resources and strengths, both personal and in their social networks. • Prepare to acknowledge the changes occurring all the time. • Regard clients as resourceful and capable of change. • Before the session, think of your client at their best.

(Continued)

Table A.5 Principles of Leave No Trace for Solution-Focused Outdoor Therapy (*Cont'd*)

Leave No Trace	*Outdoor Practice*	*General Therapeutic Practice*	*Solution-Focused Practice*
Travel, Work, and Camp on Durable Surfaces	• Reduce erosion, soil damage, habitat destruction.	• Stay on the surface, not digging too deep unless it is helpful. • Do not make assumptions. • Do not give unsolicited advice.	• Work with your clients' resilience, strengths, and instances of coping well. • Clients' solutions are more likely to fit their particular situation and are more likely to be implemented and maintained. • Work with what works well. • Understand what your client wants from the session. • Work with your client to navigate to their preferred future, or the destination for the session.

Dispose of Waste Properly	• Bag and take away all forms of waste in a hard leakproof container. • Do not pollute water sources. • Do not bury or burn rubbish.	• Take care not to ask careless questions and apologize for the "stupid" questions. • Avoid "diagnosing" your client through the lens of your own experience. • Avoid countertransference and prescribing "solutions" from one's own narrative and experiences. • The client is the expert.
Leave What You Find	• Do not remove flora, fauna, or artifacts. • Do not add graffiti or carve natural surfaces. • Do not hack at vegetation unnecessarily, or throw rocks recklessly over cliffs or down steep slopes.	• Respect the client's experience and position of expert on themselves. • Maintain confidentiality. • Respect clients' knowledge and preferences of what they want from talking with you. • Do not be a tourist in clients' lives. • The client is not the problem.

(*Continued*)

Table A.5 Principles of Leave No Trace for Solution-Focused Outdoor Therapy (*Cont'd*)

Leave No Trace	Outdoor Practice	General Therapeutic Practice	Solution-Focused Practice
Minimize Campfire Impacts	• Avoid scorching the ground, take care not to set peat or grassland or forests on fire. • Use established fire pits, avoid excessive smoke, and keep fires as small as possible. • If the fire is too big, we do not know what damage we will find should we leave it unattended. • Extinguish all fires. • Tidy fire pits and replace turf if digging a fresh pit.	• Avoid re-invoking or causing further trauma. • Do not dig deep into issues you cannot extinguish before the session's end. • Avoid insensitivity and insincerity.	• Be careful giving praise, should it sound inauthentic. • Validate the client's experience and avoid prescribing your own solutions. • Problems that appear complex might not require a complex solution. • In wet weather we find dry wood within a log and focus on growing a fire from it, as we would listen for exceptions and instances of a preferred future already in existence.

Respect Wildlife	• Do not chase, intimidate, or damage fauna and flora. • Keep disturbance through noise, for example, minimal.	• Respect everything our client brings to the session. • Do not take anything away from a session without clear permission.	• Recognize everything the client brings, especially ways to survive, their determination, and perseverance. • Tread lightly, conscientiously, and with respect.
Be Considerate to Other Visitors	• Be polite and considerate to other trail users, campsite users, river access and egress points. Give way to smaller or faster groups. Keep noise to a minimum at night.	• Be considerate to other stakeholders important to our clients.	• Respect others supplying third person narratives. • Be aware of solution-forced influences.

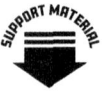

Appendix H – First Session Checklist for Practitioners

☐ Have consent forms, including routine and emergency contact numbers, medical details, been returned for each member of your group?

☐ Have you assembled all the necessary permissions, permits, tickets, bookings? Have you collected any necessary keys or lock codes?

☐ Have you read over referral notes to prepare (name of co-adventurer, age, pertinent information, etc.)? Reading over referral notes is something to be done with caution. Note behavior that could put the work at risk, such as sexualized behavior, arson, theft, absconding, anything with violence. Think how risk can be managed as you have an enhanced duty of care towards everyone involved. Remember to avoid becoming problem-focused, to think about good things associated with co-adventurers before you meet, to have options to curtail time in remote places, plan escape routes and emergency pick-up points should they be needed. Do this in the same way you would plan to escape the river, or mountain, in the event of bad weather or an accident.

☐ Have you prepared the feedback-informed treatment measures for outcome monitoring?

☐ If outdoors, have you prepared and thoroughly checked all outdoor equipment required – especially safety equipment such as ropes, karabiners, harnesses, helmets, and buoyancy aids, first aid kit, risk assessments, reviewed safety protocols, arranged call-outs with responsible people, and arranged call-ins with mentors and/or supervisors. Do the people who have agreed to be your emergency contact know what to do should you not call in? Do the people who might come out to you have a map of your route with meeting places marked on it? The time to check equipment is well before you need to use it, and in a place where replacing it is relatively straightforward. Make any damaged safety kit unusable (destroy it). First aid kits are often overlooked. Make sure they are fit for purpose then sealed so that they are waterproof, not just shower proof.

☐ Is all personal protective equipment in good condition, and fit and size appropriate? Check harnesses and buoyancy aids especially.

☐ Have you prepared spare clothes, waterproofs, comfort food, water, shelter, lighting, and phone charger equipment to be kept at the end of a journey?

☐ Paper maps are increasingly not used in preference to digital maps and location apps. Always have a paper map for the area you are working in, a working compass, and a watch.

☐ Are your co-adventurers well briefed and appropriately equipped? Is any equipment they are bringing fit for purpose? Make time for thorough pre-trip equipment checks. Take a set of weighing scales along to the pre-check meeting. No one should be carrying more than a third of their body weight. At the pre-trip check-in make sure co-adventurers bringing medication have it labeled with the owner's name, what the medication is, and the time and dosage, sealed and mentioned on their consent forms.

☐ How will co-adventurers return home at the end of their time with you, and with whom? Do you have this information recorded and available at the end of their time with you?

☐ Do you have phone numbers and locations of nearby A&E hospitals, emergency services, taxi firms, your insurance companies? Are staff familiar with call-out procedures for cave and mountain rescue, or the coast guard? Remind staff to cancel call-outs once they are safe.

☐ Is your disaster planning up to date? Are the people who will help with disaster management, media liaison, etc. properly briefed? Who do you report concerns to about young people and children at risk from, for example, self-harm, grooming, ongoing abuse etc.?

☐ Have you assembled appropriate repair kits?

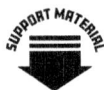

Appendix I – Guide for Expedition Reflection

This guide can be used by the expedition staff before finishing up for the day and going to sleep. Typically, we wait until our co-adventurers have returned to their tents or shelters for the night and the expedition team can enjoy a hot drink around the campfire.

Table A.6 Guide for Expedition Reflection

Climate of Competence: 1. What were you pleased to notice when the group was at its best today?
2. What was the group pleased to notice when staff were at their best today?
Planning: What clues from these events can be gathered to build on these experiences?

(Continued)

Table A.6 Guide for Expedition Reflection (*Cont'd*)

Success and Mastery: What meaning did co-adventurers derive from experiences of success and mastery that need to be noted?

Engagement: Who in the group was least engaged? Have they given any feedback that we can use to improve things for them?

Planning: What steps will be taken tomorrow to better engage the co-adventurer? Who is responsible for following this through?

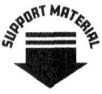

Appendix J – Solution-Focused Journal Prompts

Best Hopes Questions

- After this expedition, what would be the first thing you noticed upon returning home that told you this experience was beneficial?
  - What would [third party witness] notice that would indicate to them that changes have occurred?
- If [insert problem] was no longer an issue, what would be different?
- Your group members will know you are heading in the right direction by _____.
- What have you done to be successful during the outdoor expedition?
- Who has witnessed you at your best? What did they witness? What would they say about you?
- Suppose I was a fly on the wall when you return home. What would I notice to indicate a change has occurred?
- You described how you will know if this expedition is successful. What will I notice during the remainder of our experience that indicates you are heading in that direction?
- When were you at your best today? What difference did it make?
- What advice would you give to someone going through similar situations as you?
- What will be a sign that things are going slightly better?

Exceptions Questions

- What changes have occurred since you heard of our work together?
- What do you notice that shows you are already heading in the right direction?
  - What would you notice if you could make that happen a bit more often?
- What would [third party witness] say about your ability to make that change?
- What was different about the [how you challenged the problem]?
- What other successes have you had previously?
- If you could do that again, what would [third party witness] notice?
- When is the problem not a problem? Or when are the times you find yourself coping?
  - What would others notice?
  - What is different about those times?

Reflecting on Success and Mastery

- I noticed you were [insert experience of success and mastery] today. How were you able to do that?
- How did you manage to [insert experience of success and mastery]?
- How did you know [insert experience of success and mastery] was needed?
- Is that different from other experiences?
- You were successful in [insert experience of success and mastery]. What could you take away from that experience that you could use in other situations at home?
  - What difference will that make?
  - What will others notice?
- What strengths did you use to be successful in [insert experience of success and mastery]?
- How could you make [insert experience of success and mastery] happen more often?

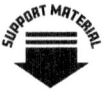

Appendix K – Solution-Focused Referral Worksheet

Table A.7 Solution-Focused Outdoor Therapy Referral Worksheet

Name of Co-Adventurer:	Date of Birth:
Name of Referrer:	Date of Referral:
Reason for referral:	
Suppose your child/client/student engages in our programs, what will you notice that indicates the program was beneficial?	
Strengths/resources assessment: What about the client should not change?	

(Continued)

Table A.7 Solution-Focused Outdoor Therapy Referral Worksheet (*Cont'd*)

What will be the first sign indicating that participation was useful?
Any risks for participation?
Referral completed by:

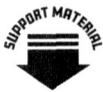

Appendix L – Solution-Focused Exercises for Parents

Many of these activities are adapted from the True North Expeditions, Inc.'s Parent Workbook and the work of other family therapy practitioners, such as Selekman and Beyebach (2013), who encourage us to view these exercises as *experiments*. They might engage those you work with, they might not. You can adapt these to the context of your work. You may invite a parent to take part in one of these activities when you drop a young one home from one of your adventures or invite parents to consider these as journal assignments while being mindful of different abilities regarding literacy.

Pretreatment Changes

- What changes, big or small, have you noticed since we spoke about your child engaging in our work?
  - What has helped these changes to happen?
  - What have you done differently?
  - What has your child done differently?

Planning the Perfect Day

We would like to invite you to write about spending the perfect day with your child. Before you reach the end, write about all the differences you noticed in how you interacted together. What are you doing differently on this perfect day? Remember that this preferred day is about the *presence* of something preferred, not what is *absent*.

Heroic Parenting

Consider the quote: "For each account of hardship there is a story of struggle, for each setback a story of perseverance, and for each misfortune a story of survival" (Ratner et al., 2012). Think about how this quote relates to your parenting journey.

- How have you managed to keep going?
- How have you prevented things from getting worse?

Resource Audit for Your Child

Take 15–20 minutes and write down every accomplishment, strength, resource, and capability your child has shown you in their life. Think about how you can help cultivate more of this in the future.

Resource Audit for Parents

- The bravest thing I've ever done is:
- My best accomplishment:
- I am at my best when:
- People know I am at my best when:
- I have learned the most about being a good parent from:
- How have my children exceeded my expectations?

Confidence Test

On a scale of 0 to 10, what is your level of confidence that the preferred future you described previously will happen (with 0 being the lowest and 10 the highest). List all the contributions to your score, let's go for 20. Which one would be the easiest to have more of, and what difference would that make?

- What gives you confidence, given what you know about yourself, that there is a chance of progressing?
- What strategies do you have for coping in the future?

Preparing for Returning Home

- Imagine that two months have passed since your child has returned from our program. How will you know that you have successfully established a new family environment?
  - What will you notice?
- Imagine it is now one month after the program. What else do you need to notice to arrive at the future you described above?
- Your child is arriving home in just a few days. What would you notice that shows you are welcoming them into a new family environment?

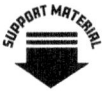

The Secret Surprise

Invite the parent to do something playful that will surprise the young person. They are instructed not to tell their child about the surprise. Instruct the child to look out for the surprise like a detective on high alert. You can also switch roles and have the child do a secret surprise for the parent(s).

Sherlock Holmes

Research has told us that parents see improvements when they set healthy and achievable boundaries (Note: With any teen, pick your battles wisely!). Adolescents want their efforts recognized and rewarded. This task is called the Sherlock Holmes assignment because we need you to be our secret detective. We want you to be on red alert looking for moments, no matter how big or small, which indicate that things are heading towards the preferred future you have described. Write a list. The longer the better. Let us know what you find over the next week.

Appendix M – 12 Keys to Proficiency in Outdoor Therapy

To reflect on your proficiencies, we recommend printing the image below. Starting with the pedagogy domain, imagine the center of the large web is a zero and the outer rim a 10. Think about this like you are asking yourself scaling questions. Rate your competence in each domain by placing a dot between the center of the large circle and the specific domain. Connect the dots with a ruler or straight edge to create a snapshot of your perceived competencies.

We recommend reflecting with your supervisor or coach, or network of peers, to develop a plan to focus on one or more of the key proficiencies worthy of further professional development.

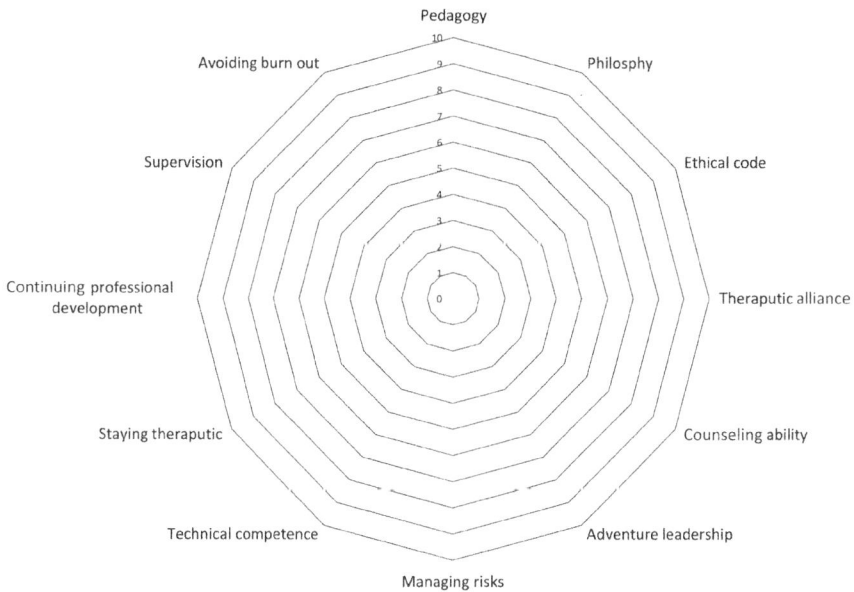

Pedagogy
10
9
8
7
6
5
4
3
2
1
0

Avoiding burn out

Philosphy

Supervision

Ethical code

Continuing professional development

Theraputic alliance

Staying theraputic

Counseling ability

Technical competence

Adventure leadership

Managing risks

Figure A.2 12 Keys to Proficiency: Characteristics of an Adventure Practitioner (Natynczuk, 2019)

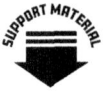

List the top three areas in need of development:

1. _____
2. _____
3. _____

In the space below, consider the following questions to help develop a plan of action.

- Who do you know who is competent with this proficiency and could help?
- What differences would you (or your co-adventurers) notice if you developed this skill further?
- You have rated this competency at [insert number] out of 10. What will be the next sign you will notice to score yourself one number higher?
- When will you make time to focus on this area of your practice?
- Who can coach you to develop this skill further?
- What systems can you implement to help you focus this skill further?
- Suppose you receive further training; how will you ensure the training has improved this specific area of development?

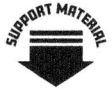

Appendix N – Feedback-Informed Treatment Measures

The following pages contain the measures and graphs we use for feedback-informed treatment. It is important, however, that you obtain your free license to utilize these tools in your practice. Contained within the free license to use these measures in your practice are instructions for using the measures and graphs with particular age groups. That said, we encourage all practitioners interested in implementing FIT in their practice to engage with the relevant literature and engage in appropriate training.

You can download the measures from: https://scott-d-miller-ph-d.myshopify.com/collections/performance-metrics/products/performance-metrics-licenses-for-the-ors-and-srs

If you are an agency, please contact Dr. Scott D. Miller at www.scottdmiller.com/

To take your feedback-informed treatment practice to the next level, we highly recommend purchasing associated software, such as MyOutcomes, FIT Outcomes, or Open FIT. More information about these programs is available on Dr. Miller's website.

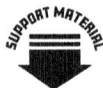

Outcome Rating Scale (ORS)

Name _____ Age (Yrs):____ Sex: M / F
Session # _____ Date: _____
Who is filling out this form? Please check one: Self_____ Other_____
If other, what is your relationship to this person? _____

Looking back over the last week (or since your last visit), including today, help us understand how you have been feeling by rating how well you have been doing in the following areas of your life, where marks to the left represent low levels and marks to the right indicate high levels. *If you are filling out this form for another person, please fill out according to how you think he or she is doing.*

Individually
(Personal well-being)

I--I

Interpersonally
(Family, close relationships)

I--I

Socially
(Work, school, friendships)

I--I

Overall
(General sense of well-being)

I--I

International Center for Clinical Excellence

www.centerforclinincalexcellence.com

© 2000, Scott D. Miller and Barry L. Duncan

To download free copies of these measures please register online at:
http://www.scottdmiller.com/?q=node/6

Figure A.3 Outcome Rating Scale

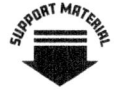

Session Rating Scale (SRS V.3.0)

Name _____ Age (Yrs):____
ID# _____ Sex: M / F
Session # _____ Date: _____

Please rate today s session by placing a mark on the line nearest to the description that best
fits your experience.

Relationship

I did not feel heard,
understood, and
respected.

I---I

I felt heard,
understood, and
respected.

Goals and Topics

We did *not* work on or
talk about what I
wanted to work on and
talk about.

I---I

We worked on and
talked about what I
wanted to work on and
talk about.

Approach or Method

The therapist s
approach is not a good
fit for me.

I---I

The therapist s
approach is a good fit
for me.

Overall

There was something
missing in the session
today.

I---I

Overall, today s
session was right for
me.

International Center for Clinical Excellence

www.centerforclinincalexcellence.com

© 2002, Scott D. Miller, Barry L. Duncan, & Lynn Johnson

Figure A.4 Session Rating Scale

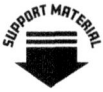

Child Outcome Rating Scale (CORS)

Name _____ Age (Yrs): _____
Sex: M / F _____
Session # _____ Date: _____
Who is filling out this form? Please check one: Child_____ Caretaker_____
  If caretaker, what is your relationship to this child? _____

How are you doing? How are things going in your life? Please make a mark on the scale to let us know. The closer to the smiley face, the better things are. The closer to the frowny face, things are not so good. *If you are a caretaker filling out this form, please fill out according to how you think the child is doing.*

Me
(How am I doing?)

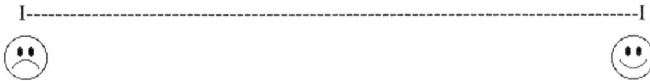

I---I

Family
(How are things in my family?)

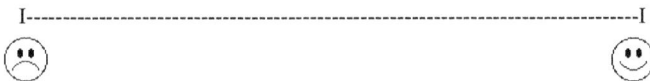

I---I

School
(How am I doing at school?)

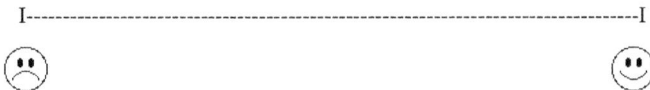

I---I

Everything
(How is everything going?)

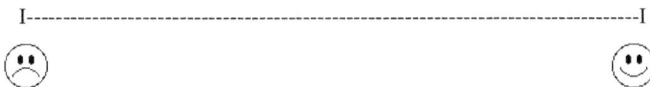

I---I

International Center for Clinical Excellence

www.centerforclinincalexcellence.com

© 2003, Barry L. Duncan, Scott D. Miller, & Jacqueline A. Sparks

To download free copies of these measures please register online at:
http://www.scottdmiller.com/?q=node/6

Figure A.5 Child Outcome Rating Scale

Child Session Rating Scale (CSRS)

Name _____ Age (Yrs): ____
Sex: M / F
Session # ____ Date: _____

How was our time together today? Please put a mark on the lines below to let us know how you feel.

Listening

did not always
listen to me.

I---I

listened to me.

How Important

What we did and
talked about was not
really that important
to me.

I---I

What we did and
talked about were
important to me.

What We Did

I did not like
what we did
today.

I---I

I liked what
we did
today.

Overall

I wish we could do
something different.

I---I

I hope we do the
same kind of
things next time.

International Center for Clinical Excellence

www.centerforclinincalexcellence.com

© 2003, Barry L. Duncan, Scott D. Miller, Jacqueline A. Sparks

To download free copies of these measures please register online at
http://www.scottdmiller.com/?q=node/6

Figure A.6 Child Session Rating Scale

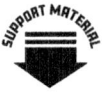

Young Child Outcome Rating Scale (YCORS)

Name _____ Age (Yrs):____
Sex: M / F____
Session # ____ Date: _____

Choose one of the faces that shows how things are going for you. Or, you can draw one
below that is just right for you.

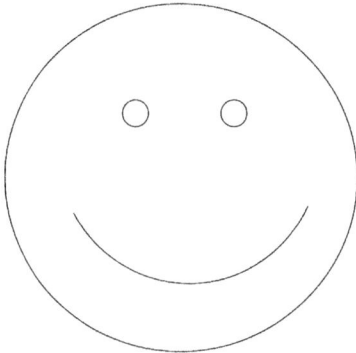

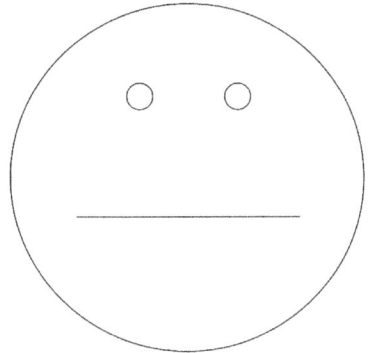

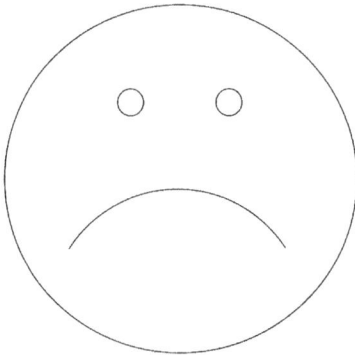

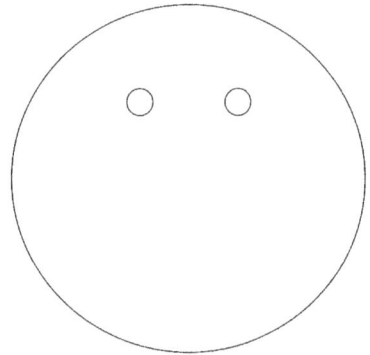

International Center for Clinical Excellence

www.centerforclinincalexcellence.com

© 2003, Barry L. Duncan, Scott D. Miller, Andy Huggins, and Jacqueline A. Sparks

To download free copies of these measures please register online at:
http://www.scottdmiller.com/?q=node/6

Figure A.7 Young Child Outcome Rating Scale

Young Child Session Rating Scale (YCSRS)

Name _____ Age (Yrs):____
Sex: M / F_____
Session # ____ Date: _____

Choose one of the faces that shows how it was for you to be here today. Or, you can draw one below that is just right for you.

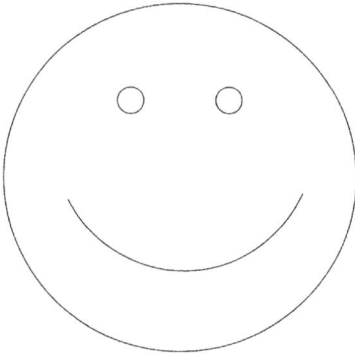

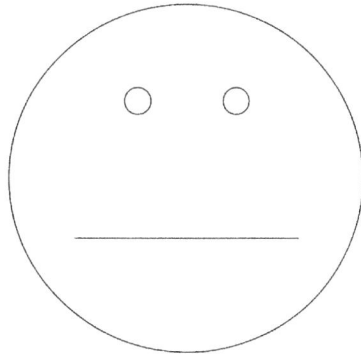

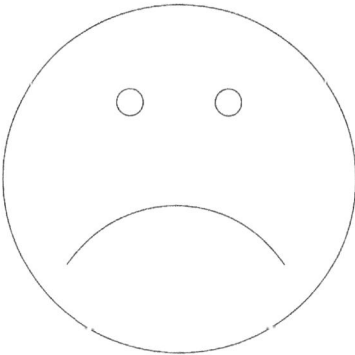

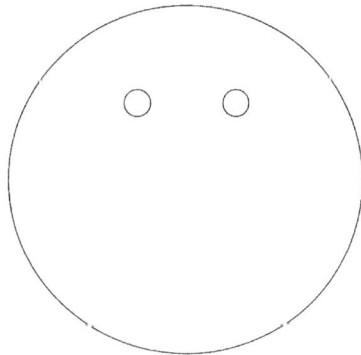

International Center for Clinical Excellence

www.centerforclinicalexcellence.com
© 2003, Barry L. Duncan, Scott D. Miller, Andy Huggins, & Jacqueline Sparks

To download free copies of these measures please register online at:
http://www.scottdmiller.com/?q=node/6

Figure A.8 Young Child Outcome Rating Scale

Copyright material from Scott Miller (2023), *Solution-Focused Practice in Outdoor Therapy*

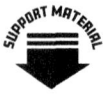

ORS/SRS - Adult

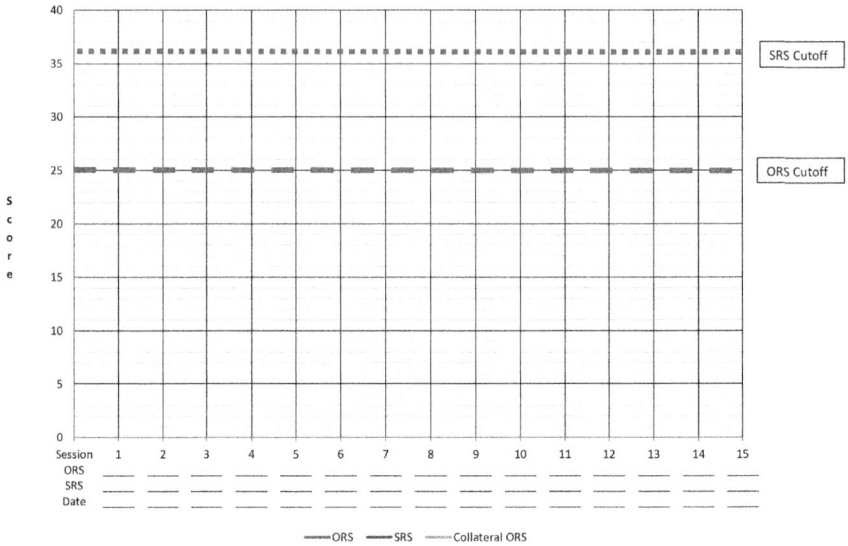

Figure A.9 Adult ORS/SRS Graph

ORS/SRS - Youth

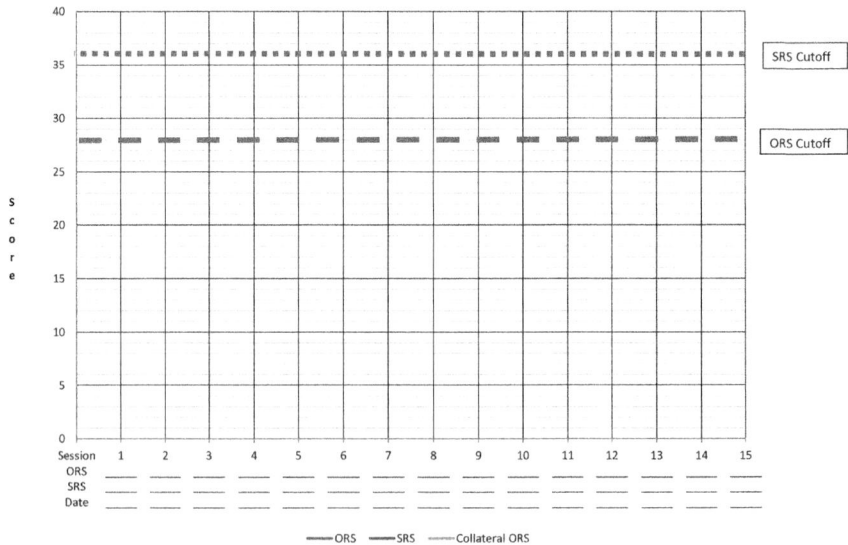

Figure A.10 Youth ORS/SRS Graph

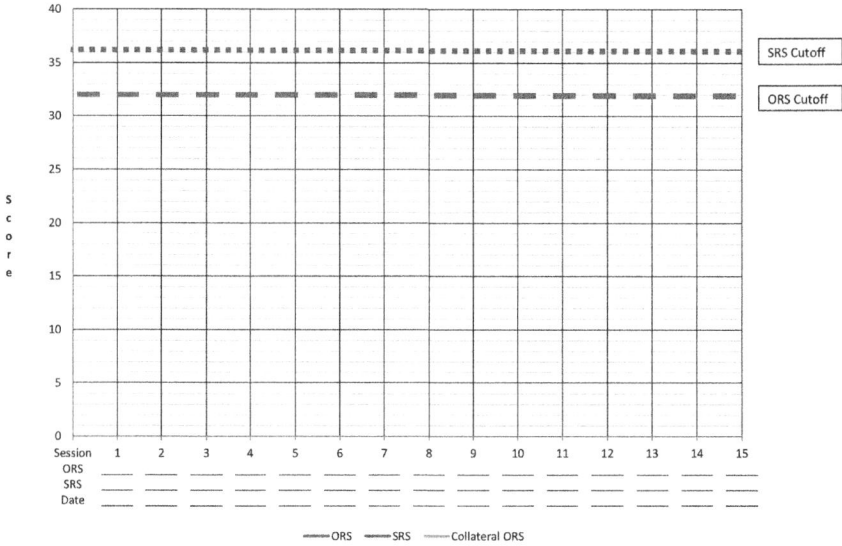

ORS/SRS - Child

Figure A.11 Young Child ORS/SRS Graph

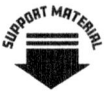

Appendix O – Interpreting Outcomes and Alliance Measures

Below are considerations for how to interpret various patterns when implementing feedback-informed treatment in the field. These considerations are informed by the work of Maeschalck and Barfknecht (2017).

Table A.8 Guide for Interpreting Outcome and Alliance Measures

Bleeding	• Evidenced by the client's outcome rating slowly decreasing. • If no change occurs within a couple of sessions, consider changes to the approach you are using. • Explore the alliance in more detail with the client. • Inquire if your work is matching client preferences.
Dipping	• Evidenced by a rapid drop on the outcome rating. • This typically means something has occurred outside of the therapeutic interaction (extratherapeutic factor). • Inquire with the client about what led to the rapid decrease. • Monitor closely until the issue is resolved. • Remind the client that the outcome measure should relate to the purpose of your work together and how things have gone, on average, since your previous administration of the measure.

(Continued)

Table A.8 Guide for Interpreting Outcome and Alliance Measures (*Cont'd*)

Seesawing or Fluctuating Scores	• Evidenced by outcome rating scores fluctuating up and down between high/low levels of distress. • This may reflect instability in the client's life, but more than likely is an indication they are completing the measure based on how they feel at this very moment. • Ensure your client understands how to complete the measure. • If the seesawing is related to instability, tailor your approach to assist the client, maybe increasing the frequency of your sessions.
Plateauing Scores	• Evidenced by a lack of progress after a couple of sessions but after previous progress. • Discuss strategies for maintaining and consolidating the gains made. • If you continue seeing the client too frequently, the client's score may begin to fluctuate as the reason that brought the client to therapy has improved but they are now reflecting the normal ups and downs of everyday life. • Spread out your sessions.

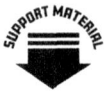

Appendix P – Progress Report

This document should be completed together with a co-adventurer. On an expedition or residential setting, we want to do this at a minimum once a week or maximum every three days.

Table A.9 Feedback-Informed Outdoor Therapy Progress Report

Co-adventurer name:	Date:
Practitioner name:	Session number:
Progress: [ ] Better [ ] Same [ ] Worse	ORS score:
How was progress addressed?	
What is the plan for in between sessions?	
How does the co-adventurer view the relationship?	
If the practitioner were to do that session over again, what should they do differently?	
Co-adventurer signature:	
Practitioner signature:	

Appendix Q – Feedback-Informed Supervision Table

Table A.10 Case Presentation Template for Feedback-Informed Supervision

Case Presentation	
Name:	Age:
Gender identity:	
Relationship/family:	
Work/education:	
Treatment start:	Current treatment:
Previous treatment:	
Abuse:	
Reasons for seeking treatment:	
Outcome Data	
First ORS score:	Last ORS score:
Quality of the Therapeutic Alliance	
First SRS score:	Last SRS score:
Relational bond:	
Best hopes/purpose:	
Means/methods:	

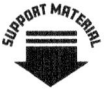

Appendix R – Format for Evidence-Informed Supervision Outdoors

Table A.11 Format for Evidence-Informed Supervision Outdoors

Practitioner's name:	Date:
Who is present in the meeting?	
Presenting problem (only discuss issues relating to a lack of progress or engagement):	
Do you have data relating the co-adventurer's outcomes? [ ] Yes [ ] No	
Have you sought client feedback relating to this issue? [ ] Yes [ ] No	
If so, describe what the data indicate.	

(Continued)

Table A.11 Format for Evidence-Informed Supervision Outdoors (*Cont'd*)

What is the co-adventurer's view of the therapeutic relationship?
What does the client want from your work together?
Given this information, what actionable steps can you take to utilize the data and client voice to improve service delivery?

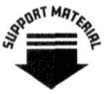

Appendix S – Questions for Solution-Focused Supervision

These are questions that should inform the supervisor-practitioner relationship before supervision begins. This page is based on an exercise from BRIEF http://www.brief.org.uk/ (www.brief.org.uk).

- How will you know that you are getting what you want from supervision?
- How will I know that this supervision is useful for you?
- Suppose we have been meeting for a few months, what else would tell you it is being useful?
- How have you made supervision useful in the past?
- What do I need to know about your way of working?
- How will you know that your way of working is moving forward?
- What kind of cases/situations/problems are you good at working with?
- What would your clients say about your way of working?
- What would your clients notice about your work as it moves forward?
- If I were to feel anxious about what I was hearing about a particular case, how would you like us to handle that situation?
- At the end of the interview, give constructive feedback on whatever skills and expectations you have been impressed by.

Appendix T – Striving for Excellence

Table A.12 Template for Building a Culture of Excellence

Start of the Week	*End of the Week*
Write your thoughts for how you will be a better practitioner this week. Only one to two sentences.	*Capture your weekly learnings. What were your shortcomings? Where could you have improved? One to two sentences.*

(Continued)

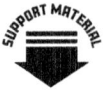

Table A.12 Template for Building a Culture of Excellence (*Cont'd*)

Index

Printed in Great Britain
by Amazon

51956947R00170